Anti-Inflammatory DIET COOKBOOK

Solving Inflammation Challenges with Ease and Delight - Based on Insights from 3,000 Interviews, Meal Plans, FAQ, and More

CLAIRE SMITH

Claire Smith

Copyright © 2023 by Claire Smith. All rights reserved.

No part of this publication may be reproduced, distributed, or transmitted in any form or by any means, including photocopying, recording, or other electronic or mechanical methods, without the prior written permission of the publisher, except in the case of brief quotations embodied in critical reviews and certain other noncommercial uses permitted by copyright law.

The information contained in this book is based on the author's research, experience, and expertise, and is intended to provide helpful and informative material on the subject matter covered.

However, the author and publisher cannot guarantee the accuracy, completeness, or reliability of the information presented, and disclaim any liability for any damages or losses that may result from the use of this information.

The trademarks mentioned in this book are for clarification purposes only, and are the property of their respective owners.

The use of these trademarks does not imply endorsement or affiliation with the author or publisher, nor does it imply any commercial relationship with these companies.

This book is the sole property of the author, and any unauthorized use or distribution is strictly prohibited.

Any violation of this copyright will result in legal action. Thank you for respecting the hard work and dedication of the author.

Table of Contents

INTRODUCTION 7
    Overview of The Anti-Inflammatory Diet 7
    Importance of Nutrition in Reducing Inflammation 7
    Tips for Incorporating Anti-Inflammatory Foods into Daily Life 8

CHAPTER 1. UNDERSTANDING INFLAMMATION AND ANTI-INFLAMMATORY APPROACHES 10
    Chronic Inflammation and Its Impact on Health 10
    Health Conditions Linked to Inflammation 10
    Benefits of An Anti-Inflammatory Diet 11
    Best Natural Anti-Inflammatory Herbs and Spices 13
    Supplements That Actually Work 13
    Autoimmune Protocol (AIP) 14
    Natural Alternatives to NSAIDs 15
    What to Avoid 16

CHAPTER 2. BREAKFAST AND BRUNCH RECIPES 17
    1. Oatmeal Pancakes 18
    2. Overnight Coconut Chia Oats 18
    3. Seared Syrupy Sage Pork Patties 19
    4. Spinach Frittata 19
    5. Buckwheat Crêpes with Berries 20
    6. Turkey with Thyme and Sage Sausage 20
    7. Buckwheat Waffles 21
    8. Smoked Salmon Scrambled Eggs 21
    9. Cucumber Bites 22
    10. Yogurt, Berry, and Walnut Parfait 22
    11. Spiced Popcorn 23
    12. Poached Eggs 23
    13. Plum, Pear and Berry-Baked Brown Rice 24
    14. Spiced Morning Chia Pudding 24
    15. Overnight Muesli 25
    16. Gingerbread Oatmeal 25
    17. Spinach Fritters 26
    18. Mushroom and Bell Pepper Omelet 26
    19. Warm Chia-Berry Non-dairy Yogurt 27
    20. Chia Breakfast Pudding 27
    21. Coconut Pancakes 28

CHAPTER 3. SOUPS AND SALADS RECIPES 29
    22. Golden Mushroom Soup 29
    23. Lime Spinach and Chickpeas Salad 30
    24. Brown Rice and Chicken Soup 31
    25. Lentils and Turmeric Soup 31
    26. Garbanzo and Kidney Bean Salad 32
    27. Avocado Side Salad 32
    28. Coconut Cashew Soup with Butternut Squash 33
    29. Beef & Vegetable Soup 33
    30. Persimmon Salad 34
    31. Italian Wedding Soup 34
    32. Spicy Pumpkin Soup 35

33. STUFFED PEPPER SOUP 35
34. WHEATBERRY SALAD 36
35. ORANGE SOUP 36
36. CHIPOTLE SQUASH SOUP 37
37. SOUTHWESTERN BEAN-AND-PEPPER SALAD 37
38. CHICKEN NOODLE SOUP 38
39. ROASTED CARROT SOUP 38
40. CHOPPED TUNA SALAD 39
41. CHICKEN SQUASH SOUP 39
42. FENNEL PEAR SOUP 40
43. NUTTY AND FRUITY GARDEN SALAD 40
44. COUSCOUS SALAD 41
45. SHOEPEG CORN SALAD 41

CHAPTER 4.   MAIN COURSE RECIPES 42

MEAT-BASED RECIPES 42
46. PORK WITH OLIVES 43
47. PORK WITH THYME SWEET POTATOES 43
48. PORK KABOBS WITH BELL PEPPERS 44
49. SPICED GROUND BEEF 44
50. MUSTARD PORK MIX 44
51. BEEF WITH CARROT & BROCCOLI 46
52. CRISPY BEEF CARNITAS 46
53. CRANBERRY PORK 46
54. OREGANO PORK 48
55. PORK WITH CHILI ZUCCHINIS AND TOMATOES 48

POULTRY-BASED RECIPES 49
56. CHICKEN LETTUCE CUPS 50
57. CHICKEN WITH COCONUT MILK 50
58. EASY TURKEY LETTUCE WRAPS 51
59. CHICKEN WITH SNOW PEAS AND BROWN RICE 51
60. ORANGE CHICKEN LEGS 52
61. TURKEY SAUSAGES 52
62. ROSEMARY CHICKEN 53
63. CINNAMON CHICKEN PESTO PASTA 53
64. ROASTED CHICKEN 54

FISH-BASED RECIPES 55
65. SEARED GARLICKY COCONUT SCALLOPS 56
66. HONEY SCALLOPS 56
67. GARLIC COD MEAL 57
68. SAUTÉ LEMON-CAPER TROUT 57
69. FRESH MUSSELS IN COCONUT HERB BROTH 58
70. CABBAGE WITH ANCHOVIES 58
71. COCONUT CHILI SALMON 59
72. KALE COD SECRET 59
73. SALMON BROCCOLI BOWL 60
74. HERBED MUSSELS TREAT 60
75. AHI POKE WITH CUCUMBER 62
76. SOUP OF OYSTERS AND MUSHROOMS 61
77. FISH STICKS WITH AVOCADO DIPPING SAUCE 61
78. COCONUT-CRUSTED SHRIMP 62

VEGETARIAN RECIPES 64
79. GINGER CARROT AND PINEAPPLE JUICE 65
80. BUCKWHEAT LEMON TABBOULEH 65

- 81. Sauté Lentil Sloppy Joes ... 66
- 82. Pesto Portobello Mushroom Burger ... 66
- 83. Fresh Spring Roll Wraps ... 67
- 84. Stir-Fried Squash ... 67
- 85. Mushroom Tacos ... 68
- 86. Curried Okra ... 68
- 87. Turmeric Endives ... 69
- 88. Cauliflower Hash Brown ... 69
- 89. Roasted Seasoned Carrots ... 70
- 90. Braised Kale ... 70
- 91. Sweet Potato Puree ... 71

VEGAN RECIPES ... 72
- 92. Cauliflower Mashed Potatoes ... 73
- 93. Paprika Brussels Sprouts ... 73
- 94. Baked Sweet Potatoes with Tomatoes ... 74
- 95. Zucchini Arugula and Olive Salad ... 75
- 96. Easy Slow Cooker Caramelized Onions ... 75
- 97. Spicy Wasabi Mayonnaise ... 76
- 98. Stir-Fried Almond and Spinach ... 76
- 99. Roasted Portobellos with Rosemary ... 76
- 100. Vegetable Potpie ... 77
- 101. Cilantro and Avocado Platter ... 77
- 102. Onion and Orange Healthy Salad ... 78
- 103. Broccoli with Garlic and Lemon ... 78

CHAPTER 5. SIDE DISHES AND ACCOMPANIMENTS RECIPES ... 79

- 104. Salt & Vinegar Kale Crisps ... 79
- 105. Chili Broccoli ... 80
- 106. Lime Carrots ... 80
- 107. Tomato Bulgur ... 81
- 108. Green Beans ... 81
- 109. Basil Olives Mix ... 82
- 110. Lemon Asparagus ... 82
- 111. Mascarpone Couscous ... 82
- 112. Balsamic Cabbage ... 83
- 113. Spiced Nuts ... 83
- 114. Parmesan Endives ... 83
- 115. Fresh Strawberry Salsa ... 84
- 116. Roasted Carrots ... 84
- 117. Beet Hummus ... 84
- 118. Celery and Fennel Salad with Cranberries ... 85
- 119. Roasted Garlic Chickpeas ... 85
- 120. Roasted Parsnips ... 85
- 121. Crispy Corn ... 86
- 122. Easy Guacamole ... 86
- 123. Lima Beans Dish ... 87
- 124. Cashew "Humus" ... 87
- 125. Apple Crisp ... 88

CHAPTER 6. SNACKS, APPETIZERS, DESSERTS, AND SWEET TREATS RECIPES ... 89

- 126. Strawberry Granita ... 89
- 127. Fragrant Honey Panna Cotta ... 90
- 128. Honey Stewed Apples ... 91
- 129. Smashed Peas with Dill and Mint ... 91

130. Mango Mug Cake 91
131. Greek Yogurt with Berries, Nuts and Honey 91
132. Chocolate Cups 92
133. Cinnamon Turmeric Golden Milk 92
134. Cherry Vanilla Ice Cream 93
135. Ruby Pears Delight 93
136. Garlicky Dill Cucumber and Yogurt Dip 93
137. Fresh Blackberry Granita with Lemon Syrup 94
138. Chickpea Paste with Onion 94
139. Chickpea and Garlic Hummus 94
140. Skewers of Tofu and Zucchini 94
141. Pear and Cinnamon Pudding 95
142. Healthy Trail Mix 95
143. Sweet Potato Muffins 96
144. Coconut Rice with Blueberries 96
145. Stone Fruit Cobbler 97
146. Whole meal Rice Pudding with Plums 97
147. Sorbet with Honey and Goji Berries 98
148. Peanut Butter Toast with Vegetables 98
149. Citrus Spinach 98
150. Coconut Vanilla Tart 99

CHAPTER 7.   30 - DAYS MEAL PLAN 100

CHAPTER 8.   FREQUENTLY ASKED QUESTIONS (FAQS) 103

CHAPTER 9.   INDEX 106

CHAPTER 10.   CONVERSION TABLE 108

CONCLUSION 110

Introduction

Overview of The Anti-Inflammatory Diet

The concept of an anti-inflammatory diet is promoted as a solution to combat inflammation in the body. It is commonly believed that all forms of inflammation are negative, but in reality, inflammation is a natural and necessary response by our immune system. When our body encounters foreign substances like bacteria, viruses, allergens, or experiences an injury, our immune cells react swiftly. Symptoms such as sneezing, coughing, pain, swelling, increased blood flow, warmth, and redness indicate that our immune system is working to repair damaged tissue or fight off invaders. As the healing process progresses, inflammation gradually diminishes.

However, when inflammation persists for an extended period and starts harming healthy cells, it creates a state of pro-inflammatory conditions. Another issue arises from genetic abnormalities that cause the immune system to continuously attack the body's own cells. The autoimmune diseases lupus, fibromyalgia, multiple sclerosis, rheumatoid arthritis, Crohn's disease, and type 1 diabetes all have the potential to cause this kind of symptom. Furthermore, an unhealthy lifestyle that is defined by an absence of activity, high stress, and a diet that is heavy in calories can promote chronic low-level inflammation across the body. This type of inflammation is referred to as metaflammation. This kind of mild inflammation doesn't typically generate any apparent symptoms; however, it could prepare the way for chronic illnesses like cardiovascular disease, non-alcoholic fatty liver disease, type 2 diabetes, Alzheimer's disease, and specific cancers including as breast and colon cancer.

To address these inflammatory conditions, anti-inflammatory diets are often recommended. These diets include various foods believed to interfere with the inflammatory process, although the exact mechanisms are not fully understood and research is inconclusive. There isn't one anti-inflammatory diet plan that is appropriate for everyone, however in overall, it stresses ingesting a wide variety of fruits, vegetables, unsaturated fats, naturally processed whole grains, tea, coffee, herbs, and spices, as well as oily fish. Many anti-inflammatory foods are already incorporated into well-known diet programs like the DASH diet and the Mediterranean diet.

A diet plan designed to reduce inflammation not only emphasizes the consumption of certain foods and food groups, but it also discourages the consumption of other items that can exacerbate the condition. These involve consuming large amounts of alcohol, meals and beverages that are too processed and high in sugar, and fatty cuts of red meat.

Importance of Nutrition in Reducing Inflammation

The role of nutrition in reducing inflammation is vital as chronic inflammation is linked to various health conditions like cardiovascular disease, diabetes, obesity, and certain cancers. Adopting a healthy, anti-inflammatory diet is key to mitigating inflammation and promoting overall well-being. Here are several ways nutrition influences inflammation:

1. **Omega-3 Fatty Acids:** Essential fats found in fatty fish (salmon, sardines), walnuts, flaxseeds, and chia seeds possess potent anti-inflammatory properties. They reduce the production of pro-inflammatory molecules and promote the synthesis of anti-inflammatory compounds in the body.

2. **Antioxidants:** Colorful fruits and vegetables (berries, leafy greens, tomatoes, peppers) are rich in antioxidants. These combat oxidative stress, a contributor to inflammation, by neutralizing harmful free radicals & protecting cells from damage.
3. **Healthy Fats:** Consumption of healthy fats like those in avocados, olive oil, and nuts helps reduce inflammation. These fats contain monounsaturated fatty acids (MUFAs) known for their anti-inflammatory effects.
4. **Fiber:** High-fiber foods such as whole grains, legumes, fruits, and vegetables are beneficial in reducing inflammation. Fiber supports a healthy gut microbiome, which modulates the immune system and inflammation.
5. **Spices and Herbs:** Certain spices and herbs possess anti-inflammatory properties. Turmeric, ginger, cinnamon, and garlic are examples that have demonstrated inflammation-reducing effects.
6. **Probiotics:** Probiotics, beneficial bacteria, contribute to a healthy gut microbiome. They improve gut health, reduce the production of pro-inflammatory molecules, and help regulate inflammation.
7. **Limiting Processed Foods:** Processed foods like sugary snacks, refined grains, and fried foods often contain unhealthy fats, added sugars, and artificial additives. These can promote inflammation and should be limited in the diet.
8. **Avoiding Trigger Foods:** Some individuals have specific food intolerances or sensitivities that trigger inflammation, such as gluten, dairy, or nightshade vegetables. Identifying and avoiding these trigger foods can help reduce inflammation in susceptible individuals.

By incorporating these dietary strategies, individuals can actively reduce inflammation and promote their overall health and well-being.

Tips for Incorporating Anti-Inflammatory Foods into Daily Life

Incorporating anti-inflammatory foods into your daily life is a great way to support your overall health. Here are some practical tips to help you include more anti-inflammatory foods in your diet:

1. Prioritize fruits and vegetables: Make it a point to include a variety of colorful fruits & vegetables in your meals. Include berries to your breakfast, have a lunch salad with leafy greens, and incorporate a mix of roasted or steamed vegetables into your dinner. Experiment with different flavors and textures to keep your meals interesting.
2. Opt for whole grains: Choose whole grains like quinoa, brown rice, oats & whole wheat bread over refined grains. These whole grains retain their fiber and nutrients, which possess anti-inflammatory properties.
3. Integrate fatty fish: Incorporate fatty fish such as salmon, mackerel, and sardines into your diet a few times a week. These types of fish are rich in omega-3 fatty acids, which have powerful anti-inflammatory effects.
4. Use healthy oils: Cook with oils that have anti-inflammatory properties, such as olive oil, avocado oil, or coconut oil. These oils contain healthy fats that can help reduce inflammation in the body.
5. Spice things up: Include spices and herbs known for their anti-inflammatory properties to your meals. Turmeric, ginger, garlic, cinnamon, and oregano are examples of ingredients with well-documented anti-inflammatory benefits. Experiment with incorporating these spices and herbs into your cooking or sprinkle them on your dishes.Snack on nuts and seeds: Keep a variety of nuts and seeds like almonds, walnuts, flaxseeds, and chia seeds on hand for a quick and healthy snack. These nuts and seeds are rich in omega-3 fatty acids and other nutrients that can help combat inflammation.

6. Include legumes: Incorporate legumes such as lentils, chickpeas, and black beans into your meals. These legumes are excellent sources of plant-based protein and fiber, and they also possess anti-inflammatory properties. Include them to soups, salads, or use them to make hummus as a flavorful and nutritious addition to your diet.
7. Replace unhealthy snacks: Swap processed snacks and sugary treats with healthier alternatives. For instance, choose fresh fruits, raw vegetables with hummus, or a handful of nuts instead of reaching for cookies or chips.
8. Opt for green tea: Drink green tea, which contains antioxidants known for their anti-inflammatory effects. Substitute sugary beverages with green tea or herbal teas to increase your intake of antioxidants.
9. Plan and prep meals in advance: Take some time each week to plan and prepare meals that incorporate anti-inflammatory foods. Having healthy meals readily available can help you stay committed to your dietary goals and make it easier to choose anti-inflammatory options.

By following these tips, you can gradually incorporate more anti-inflammatory foods into your daily routine and support your overall health and well-being.

Chapter 1. Understanding Inflammation and Anti-Inflammatory Approaches

Chronic Inflammation and Its Impact on Health

Chronic inflammation, which can endure for months to years, is a prolonged and slow form of inflammation. Its severity and impact vary depending on the underlying cause of the injury and the body's ability to repair and overcome the damage. The following factors can contribute to chronic inflammation:

1. The failure to eradicate the agent that triggers acute inflammation, which includes pathogenic organisms like Mycobacterium tuberculosis, protozoa, fungi, and other parasites which may resist the body's defenses and linger in the tissue for a long amount of time; this may result in chronic inflammation.
2. Exposure to low levels of specific irritants or foreign substances that cannot be broken down by enzymes or eliminated through phagocytosis, such as long-term inhalation of substances or industrial chemicals like silica dust.
3. Autoimmune disorders, where the immune system mistakenly recognizes the body's normal components as foreign antigens and attacks healthy tissues, leading to conditions like rheumatoid arthritis (RA) or systemic lupus erythematosus (SLE).
4. Malfunctioning of cells responsible for mediating inflammation, resulting in persistent or recurrent inflammation. This can occur in auto-inflammatory disorders like Familial Mediterranean Fever.
5. Recurrent bouts of severe inflammation in the body. On the other hand, there are circumstances in which chronic inflammation is not a result of acute inflammation but rather a separate response. This is the case in conditions such as tuberculosis and rheumatoid arthritis.
6. The onset of oxidative stress and malfunction in the mitochondria by inflammatory and pharmacological agents. This involves a rise in the synthesis of molecules including free radicals, advanced glycation end products (AGEs), crystals of uric acid (urate), oxidized lipoproteins, and homocysteine, amongst other components.

Health Conditions Linked to Inflammation

Chronic inflammation may be fatal; according to estimates, 3 out of 5 individuals lose their lives due to inflammatory disorders. There are many health risks posed by inflammation, mainly including the following.

Rheumatoid Arthritis

Let's say that inflammation makes arthritis almost unbearable. A person feels hampered in his movements, and sometimes it even hurts while talking and eating. The persistent state of swelling in the joints may result in permanent tissue damage to the patient. Patients of arthritis are therefore advised to keep this inflammation in check and continuously look for measures to control it.

Psoriasis

It is another immune-mediated disease in which the patient may suffer from large patches of inflammation over the skin. It causes redness and itchiness on the skin and typically appears on the elbows, scalp, and knees. The swelling may increase if the problem is not timely dealt with.

Asthma

Asthma is a respiratory condition in which the internal lining of the human respiratory system swells, constricts the air pathways, and leads to shortness of breath. A chronic state of asthma can even be fatal for the patients. Instant anti-inflammatory measures are required to treat this condition, but the patients are also advised to avoid consuming all such items which could trigger this reaction.

Inflammatory Bowel Disease

Also known as Crohn's disease, in this condition, the inflammation occurs inside the digestive tract and swells the internal lining of the intestines. It causes pain in bowel movements, fatigue, diarrhea, and even weightlessness. Controlling the inflammation can prevent intense pain and discomfort in this disease.

Diabetes

Inflammation can lead to insulin resistance, prediabetes, and ultimately to diabetes. The pancreatic inflammation can cause damage to the insulin-producing beta cells, eventually leading to diabetes. Diabetic patients should remain extra cautious of cell or tissue damage as their bodies may not respond well to the injuries.

Obesity

Obesity and inflammation are closely linked to one another. Cronin inflammation may result in alleviating the rate of metabolism, and it may lead to unnecessary deposition of fats. The fat cells may further contribute to more inflammation, so the cycle continues. Before it gets critical, both obesity and inflammation should be dealt with.

Heart Disease

Any obstruction in the blood flow eventually affects the functioning of the cardiac muscles. Inflammation can often constrict the blood vessels and leads to higher pressure inside. It, in turn, affects the heart and may lead to minor or permanent damages.

Benefits of An Anti-Inflammatory Diet

Choosing an anti-inflammatory diet is a good idea for our health. Anti-inflammatory foods are high in antioxidants and vitamins, which slow the inflammatory response.

An anti-inflammatory diet is not a new concept; it has been around for a while. Many people have tried it and had great success. You might be surprised to learn that your favorite cuisine can cause inflammation in your body.

- Anti-inflammatory diet benefits heart health, according to a Northwestern University study, foods high in omega 3 fatty acids, such as fish, nuts, and plants, can help protect the cardiovascular system from inflammation. Eating fish twice a week can thus cut the risk of developing heart disease in half.
- An anti-inflammatory diet will benefit your joints: Anti-inflammatory diets may reduce your risk of osteoporosis by protecting your joints. The explanation is that omega-3 fatty acids can help keep your bones healthy and strong. Furthermore, according to the National Osteoporosis Foundation, anti-inflammatory diets contain antioxidants that can aid in the fight against this condition.

- An anti-inflammatory diet will benefit your gut: A common question is, "Why does my stomach hurt?" If you have irritable bowel syndrome (IBS) or pouchitis, foods high in fiber and anti-inflammatory chemicals, such as fruits, vegetables, and whole grains, may help relieve your discomfort.
- Following an anti-inflammatory diet may help you avoid becoming obese. An anti-inflammatory diet warns against overeating, which can lead to fat tissue buildup and obesity.
- Obesity and an inflammatory diet may be related in a variety of ways. Consuming more refined carbohydrates, processed meats, and junk food is one inflammatory diet. Because these meals are low in calories and fiber, a person will have to eat more to compensate for the calorie deficit and lack of satiety. Two, someone who consumes an inflammatory diet may spend more time indoors, encouraging them to consume more calories while moving less.
- People who are already suffering from inflammatory disorders may benefit from an anti-inflammatory diet in particular. Anti-inflammatory diets, for example, that exclude refined sugars and carbohydrates, may result in type 2 diabetes, metabolic syndrome, and obesity. An anti-inflammatory diet instead suggests eating whole grains like brown rice, which is high in fiber and has a low glycemic index.
- An anti-inflammatory diet may also aid in fatigue. The inflammation indicates that the immune system is functioning properly. When the immune system is completely dedicated, histamine levels rise, making a person sleepy, tired, and cranky. The immune system's activities are supposed to make you tired, allowing your body to slow down and conserve energy. Fatigue is also thought to promote rest and healing rather than limiting the body further. An anti-inflammatory diet helps to reduce or eliminate inflammation, which reduces or eliminates the fatigue-causing effects of the immune system.
- An anti-inflammatory diet that has nothing to do with obesity may aid in weight loss. Even if you are not obese, you may be overweight or on the verge of becoming obese. The high consumption of refined carbs and sugars is blamed for unintentional weight gain and other non-dietary reasons, such as sedentary lifestyles. Refined carbohydrate foods are low in nutrients, requiring more calories than necessary to meet calorie requirements.
- An anti-inflammatory diet may aid in your sleep. Diet may contribute to poor sleep quality or an inconsistent sleep pattern in a variety of ways. When you eat an inflammatory diet, you will have difficulty sleeping on a regular basis, and when you do, it will be of poor quality. An inflammatory diet can cause eating issues, such as waking up in the middle of the night to eat, which can disrupt the quality and length of sleep. Due to fatigue, you may require frequent episodes of brief sleeping, which will disrupt your night's sleep. Fortunately, an anti-inflammatory diet can help you sleep better by lowering inflammation and ensuring that your meals are calorie and mineral balanced.
- The biggest benefit of following an anti-inflammatory diet is that it can help reduce your risk of heart disease. Studies have shown that people who follow an anti-inflammatory diet are significantly less likely to develop heart disease than those who don't. Why is this? Well, an anti-inflammatory diet helps reduce the inflammation in your body, which is linked with the development of heart disease.

Best Natural Anti-Inflammatory Herbs and Spices

There are numerous natural herbs and spices renowned for their anti-inflammatory properties. Including these in your diet can potentially reduce inflammation within the body. Below are some of the most effective natural herbs and spices with anti-inflammatory benefits:

1. Turmeric: Turmeric contains curcumin, an active compound with strong anti-inflammatory properties. Curcumin effectively reduces inflammation by suppressing the production of inflammatory molecules in the body.
2. Ginger: Ginger contains gingerols, which have strong anti-inflammatory effects. It is commonly used to alleviate symptoms of arthritis and other inflammatory conditions.
3. Garlic: Garlic possesses sulfur compounds that have demonstrated anti-inflammatory properties. It can help diminish inflammation while boosting the immune system.
4. Cinnamon: Cinnamon is rich in antioxidants and anti-inflammatory compounds that aid in reducing inflammation and lowering the risk of chronic diseases.
5. Rosemary: Rosemary contains rosmarinic acid, which possesses both anti-inflammatory and antioxidant effects. It can be used as a spice or brewed into tea.
6. Sage: Sage has long been valued for its medicinal properties, including its anti-inflammatory effects. It contains rosmarinic acid, which assists in reducing inflammation within the body.
7. Cloves: Cloves contain eugenol, a compound known for its anti-inflammatory and analgesic properties. They can be added to dishes or used in tea preparations.
8. Cayenne pepper: Cayenne pepper possesses capsaicin, a compound known for its anti-inflammatory properties. It has been demonstrated to help relieve pain and diminish inflammation.
9. Black pepper: Black pepper contains piperine, a compound that has been found to possess anti-inflammatory properties. It can enhance the absorption of curcumin from turmeric.
10. Green tea: Green tea contains catechins, which are antioxidants known for their anti-inflammatory properties. Incorporating green tea into your regular diet can help reduce inflammation and support your overall well-being.

Supplements That Actually Work

Here are 10 supplements that have been shown in research to potentially help reduce inflammation. Let's take a look at each one:

Curcumin

Curcumin is a compound found in turmeric, known for its bright yellow color and commonly used in Indian cuisine. It has been found to decrease inflammation in conditions like diabetes, heart disease, inflammatory bowel disease, cancer, osteoarthritis, and rheumatoid arthritis.

Fish oil

Fish oil supplements contain omega-3 fatty acids, known for their anti-inflammatory effects. They have been studied for their potential in reducing inflammation associated with conditions like diabetes and heart disease. The primary beneficial omega-3s found in fish oil are EPA and DHA.

Ginger

Ginger possesses anti-inflammatory properties and has demonstrated the ability to reduce inflammation linked to type 2 diabetes. It may also have a positive impact on blood sugar control and inflammation levels.

Resveratrol, an antioxidant found in fruits like grapes and blueberries, has been investigated for its potential anti-inflammatory effects in conditions such as liver disease, obesity, and ulcerative colitis. Studies have shown that resveratrol supplements can improve quality of life, symptoms, and inflammation.

Spirulina

Spirulina, a type of blue-green algae, is abundant in antioxidants and has been found to reduce inflammation, support healthy aging, and potentially enhance the immune system. It may improve inflammatory markers, anemia, and immune function.

Vitamin D

These plays a critical role in immune health and possesses potent anti-inflammatory properties. Inadequate levels of vitamin D have been associated with inflammation, and supplementation has been shown to decrease inflammation in conditions like premenstrual syndrome and obesity.

Bromelain

Bromelain, a powerful enzyme found in pineapple, exhibits anti-inflammatory effects similar to nonsteroidal anti-inflammatory drugs (NSAIDs). Although research on humans is limited, bromelain has demonstrated usefulness in reducing postoperative inflammation.

Green tea extract

Green tea extract is rich in compounds like EGCG, which have anti-inflammatory properties. It has been found to significantly reduce inflammation when combined with exercise in overweight individuals.

Garlic

Garlic contains allicin, a potent anti-inflammatory compound that may also strengthen the immune system. Supplementation with aged garlic extract has shown improvements in inflammatory markers, suggesting it may reduce the risk of inflammation-related chronic diseases.

Vitamin C

These is an essential vitamin with antioxidant properties that can neutralize free radicals and reduce inflammation. It supports the immune system and may help regulate inflammation. High doses are often given intravenously in severe respiratory illnesses.

While these supplements have demonstrated potential in reducing inflammation, it's important to note that individual responses may vary. Consulting with a healthcare professional before initiating any new supplement regimen is always advisable. Additionally, focusing on meeting nutrient needs through a well-balanced diet rich in fruits, vegetables, whole grains & healthy fats should be the primary approach to reducing inflammation.

Autoimmune Protocol (AIP)

The Autoimmune Protocol, sometimes known as AIP, is an integrative method for the management of chronic disorders. It places an emphasis on supplying the body with the essential nutrients for immunological modulation, gastrointestinal health, hormone regulation, and tissue healing while simultaneously removing inflammatory irritants from the lifestyle and the diet. The AIP diet places an emphasis on having a well-rounded and comprehensive nutritional intake while discouraging the consumption of processed and refined foods. Furthermore, the AIP way of life emphasizes getting enough sleep, learning how to handle stress effectively, and engaging in regular physical activity as critical components in the process of modifying the immune system. Foods can be classified into two categories: those that promote health (nutrients) and those that undermine health (inflammatory compounds). While some foods have both health-promoting and potentially detrimental compounds, the AIP places greater emphasis on nutrient-dense foods such as organ meat, seafood &

vegetables. It excludes foods like nightshades, eggs, nuts, seeds, and alcohol that are recommended by other healthy diets but include components which could stimulate the immune system or disrupt the environment of the gut. These substances may cause inflammation. The objective is to provide the body with an abundance of nutrients while eliminating any items that can aggravate the condition being treated or slow down the recovery process.

The AIP is initially an elimination diet, removing the foods most likely to impede health. After a period of time, certain excluded foods can be reintroduced, especially those that have nutritional benefits despite potentially detrimental compounds. The AIP is not a permanent restriction but a toolbox for understanding individual reactions to food, lifestyle, and the environment, providing strategies for healing based on individual health challenges.

Beyond diet, the AIP takes a holistic approach to health, considering lifestyle factors that significantly impact immune function, gut health, and hormone regulation. Adequate sleep, stress management, and an active lifestyle are crucial for maintaining a healthy gut microbiome, supporting probiotic strains, and reducing intestinal permeability. These lifestyle factors also affect hormone modulation, insulin sensitivity, and immune function. Inflammation can be triggered by insufficient sleep, chronic stress, sedentary behavior, and overtraining. Additionally, a strong sense of connection, spending time in natural environments, and a supportive community contribute to a healthier immune system.

The AIP is supported by clinical trial evidence and draws on insights from numerous scientific studies. Studies have shown significant improvements in disease activity and health-related quality of life in patients with inflammatory bowel disease and Hashimoto's thyroiditis following the AIP. The Wahls Protocol, which shares similarities with the AIP, has also shown promising results in managing multiple sclerosis.

The growing recommendation of the AIP by clinicians, particularly in functional and integrative medicine, further supports its efficacy. Ongoing clinical research is being conducted to quantify the benefits of the AIP in specific autoimmune diseases, further highlighting the importance of diet and lifestyle as a primary course of treatment.

Natural Alternatives to NSAIDs

Research findings from as early as 1995 indicate that long-term use of non-steroidal anti-inflammatory drugs (NSAIDs) can have certain effects on the body. These effects include increasing osteoarthritis within 180 days to one year of use, interfering with tendon and tissue healing, interfering with fracture and surgical fusion healing, and increasing fracture risk. However, there are natural anti-inflammatory options available that have been used for centuries and have shown effectiveness and other health benefits.

Bromelain, derived from the pineapple plant, is a well-known anti-inflammatory agent. It contains sulfur-containing enzymes that aid in protein digestion. Bromelain has been extensively studied for its therapeutic applications, particularly in cases of injury, sprains, strains, and arthritis. It breaks down excessive fibrotic tissue after tissue healing has occurred. Fresh pineapple or bromelain supplements can be used to obtain its benefits, with typical dosages ranging from 250 to 500 milligrams three times a day. People taking certain medications should use bromelain under medical supervision.

Capsicum, found in cayenne pepper, is another beneficial anti-inflammatory agent. Topical preparations containing capsaicin, derived from capsicum, can provide relief for various conditions, including pain disorders and arthritis. Cayenne pepper has also shown positive effects on the cardiovascular system and gastrointestinal function. Spicy foods containing cayenne pepper do not cause ulcers in normal individuals. Capsaicin is available in concentrated capsule forms as well.

Curcumin, found in turmeric, has been used in Ayurvedic medicine for its anti-inflammatory properties. It has demonstrated effectiveness in treating acute inflammation and shows potential therapeutic effects against various diseases. Turmeric should be included liberally in the diet, and curcumin supplements are available. Standard dosages range from 400 to 600 milligrams three times a day.

Ginger, known for its anti-inflammatory and analgesic effects, has also shown benefits in lowering cholesterol and improving gastrointestinal function. Recommended dosage ranges from two to four grams of dry powdered ginger per day.

Other herbal options include boswellia and gugulipid, which have significant anti-inflammatory action and have been studied for treating arthritis. Boswellia and curcumin combinations have shown positive results. **Corydalis yanhusuo**, a tuber used in Chinese herbal medicine, has demonstrated anti-inflammatory activity. **Homeopathic remedies**, such as **Traumeel and Zeel**, have also been used for inflammation and pain relief.

These natural alternatives can be incorporated into daily food choices. If higher concentrations are required, over-the-counter strengths and combinations can be found in health food stores. It's important to note that homeopathy has its own principles and controversies within the scientific community.

What to Avoid

Certain foods have the ability to decrease inflammation, while others have the potential to increase inflammation within your body. Examples of foods that can exacerbate inflammation include:

- Red meats such as steak and burgers.
- Processed meats like bacon, hot dogs, and sausages.
- Foods containing white flour, like white bread, bagels, and white pasta.
- Sweet baked goods including cookies, donuts, and cakes.
- Packaged salty snacks like chips or crackers.
- Frozen dinners and ready-to-eat meals.
- Sweetened beverages like soda.
- Fried foods like French fries, fried fish, and fried chicken.
- Margarine, soybean oil, corn oil, cottonseed oil, and highly processed foods made with these oils.

Occasionally consuming small amounts of these foods might not be harmful. However, consuming them frequently can trigger inflammation due to their high content of:

- Saturated fats.
- Refined (white) carbohydrates, such as white rice.
- Excessive salt and added sugar.
- Artificial preservatives, flavors, colors, and other additives.

After some time, your immune system may come to recognize these undesirable components as toxins, which can be hazardous to your health if you continue to be exposed to them. An bad diet can trigger an inflammatory reaction, much like a physical injury or an infectious disease might.

Adopting an anti-inflammatory diet is an effective means of reducing the risk of chronic diseases. It is also recommended as a component of your overall strategy for managing existing chronic conditions.

If changing your diet seems overwhelming, consider seeking the assistance of a registered dietitian. They can guide you in making gradual modifications, enabling you to develop healthier habits over time.

Chapter 2. Breakfast and Brunch Recipes

1. Oatmeal Pancakes 18
2. Overnight Coconut Chia Oats 18
3. Seared Syrupy Sage Pork Patties 19
4. Spinach Frittata 19
5. Buckwheat Crêpes with Berries 20
6. Turkey with Thyme and Sage Sausage 20
7. Buckwheat Waffles 21
8. Smoked Salmon Scrambled Eggs 21
9. Cucumber Bites 22
10. Yogurt, Berry, and Walnut Parfait 22
11. Spiced Popcorn 23
12. Poached Eggs 23
13. Plum, Pear and Berry-Baked Brown Rice 24
14. Spiced Morning Chia Pudding 24
15. Overnight Muesli 25
16. Gingerbread Oatmeal 25
17. Spinach Fritters 26
18. Mushroom and Bell Pepper Omelet 26
19. Warm Chia-Berry Non-dairy Yogurt 27
20. Chia Breakfast Pudding 27
21. Coconut Pancakes 28

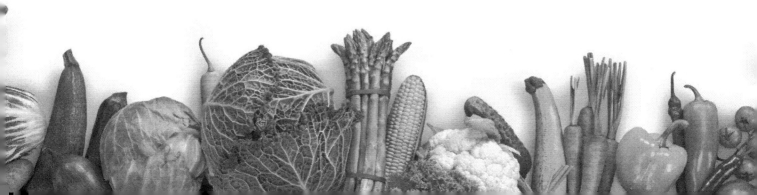

1. Oatmeal Pancakes

Preparation time: ten mins
Cooking time: twenty-five mins
Servings: 2
Ingredients:

- one and half teacups rolled oats, whole-grain
- 2 eggs, large & pastured
- 2 tsp. baking powder
- 1 banana, ripe
- 2 tbsp. water
- ¼ cup maple syrup
- one tsp. vanilla extract
- two tbsps extra virgin olive oil

Directions:

1. To form this delightful breakfast dish, you need to first blend all the ingredients in a high-speed mixer for a minute or two or till you get an even batter. Tip: To blend easily, pour egg, banana, and all other liquid ingredients first and finally add oats at the end.
2. Now, take a large skillet and warm it at medium-low temp.
3. Once the skillet is hot, ¼ cup of the batter into it and cook it for three-four mins per side or till bubbles start appearing in the middle portion.
4. Turn the pancake and cook the other side also.
5. Serve warm.

Per serving: Calories: 201kcal; Protein: 5g; Carbs: 28g; Fat: 8g

2. Overnight Coconut Chia Oats

Preparation time: ten mins
Cooking time: sixty mins
Servings: one to two
Ingredients:

- half teacup coconut milk, unsweetened
- 2 tsp. chia seeds
- one and half teacups old fashioned oats, whole grain
- half tsp. cinnamon, grounded
- 1 cup almond milk, unsweetened
- half tsp. cinnamon, grounded
- 2 tsp. date syrup
- half tsp. black pepper, grounded
- one tsp. turmeric, grounded

Directions:

1. To start with, keep the oats in the mason jar.
2. After that, mix the remaining components inside a moderate container till combined thoroughly.
3. Then, pour the solution to the jars and stir well.
4. Now, close the jar and place it in the fridge overnight.
5. In the morning, stir the solution and then enjoy it.

Per serving: Calories: 335kcal; Protein: 8g; Carbs: 34.1g; Fat: 19.9g

3. Seared Syrupy Sage Pork Patties

Preparation time: twelve mins
Cooking time: ten mins
Servings: 2
Ingredients:

- 2-lbs ground pork, pastured
- three tbsps maple syrup, grade b
- three tbsps minced fresh sage
- three-quarter tsp sea salt
- half tsp garlic powder
- one tsp solid cooking fat

Directions:

1. Break the ground pork into chunks in a mixing bowl. Drizzle evenly with the maple syrup. Sprinkle with the spices. Mix well till thoroughly combined. Form the solution into eight patties. Set aside.
2. Warm the fat in a cast-iron griddle placed at middling temp. Cook the patties for ten mins on all sides, or till browned.

Per serving: Calories: 405kcal; Protein: 30g; Carbs: 53g; Fat: 11g

4. Spinach Frittata

Preparation time: ten mins
Cooking time: twelve mins
Servings: two
Ingredients:

- two teacups of baby spinach
- one tsp of garlic powder
- two tbsps of extra-virgin olive oil
- 8 beaten eggs
- half tsp of sea salt
- two tbsps of grated parmesan cheese
- one-eighth tsp black pepper

Directions:

1. Warm up the broiler to the highest setting.
2. Warmth the olive oil in a big ovenproof griddle or pan (well-seasoned cast iron fits well) at medium-high temp. till it starts shimmering.
3. Cook, blending continuously, for around 3 minutes after introducing the spinach.
4. Whisk collectively the eggs, salt, garlic powder, and pepper inside a standard mixing cup. Carefully spill the egg solution over the spinach and cook for three mins, or till the edges of the eggs start to get established.
5. Gently raise the eggs away from the pan's sides with a rubber spatula. Enable the uncooked egg to flow into the pan's edges by tilting it. Cook for another two or three mins, just till the sides are solid.
6. Put the pan beneath the broiler and cover with the Parmesan cheese. Warm up the oven to broil for around three mins, or before the top puffs up.
7. To eat, break into wedges.

Per serving: Calories: 203kcal; Protein: 13g; Carbs: 203g; Fat: 13g

5. Buckwheat Crêpes with Berries

Preparation time: fifteen mins
Cooking time: five mins
Servings: two
Ingredients:

- half tsp of salt
- one teacup of almond milk or water
- half tsp of vanilla extract
- three tbsps of chia jam
- half teacup of buckwheat flour
- one tbsp of coconut oil (half tablespoon melted)
- 1 egg
- two teacups of fresh berries, divided

Directions:

1. Whisk collectively the salt, egg, buckwheat flour, and half tablespoon dissolved coconut oil, almond milk, and vanilla in a small mixing bowl 'til smooth.
2. Melt the remaining half tbsp of coconut oil in a wide (12-inch) non-stick griddle or pan at medium-high temp. Tilt the pan to adequately cover it in the molten oil.
3. Using a ladle in the griddle or pan, pour half a cup of batter. Tilt the pan to properly brush it with batter.
4. Cook for another two mins till the edges start to curl. Flip the crêpe with a spatula and cook for one min on the other hand. Place the crêpe on a plate and put away.
5. For the left batter, continue to make crêpe.
6. On a dish, place one crêpe, some berries, and a tbsp of Chia Jam. Cover the crêpe over the filling and seal the edges.

Per serving: Calories: 242kcal; Protein: 7g; Carbs: 33g; Fat: 11g

6. Turkey with Thyme and Sage Sausage

Preparation time: forty mins
Cooking time: twenty-five mins
Servings: 4
Ingredients:

- one lb. ground turkey
- half tsp cinnamon
- half tsp garlic powder
- one tsp fresh rosemary
- one tsp fresh thyme
- one tsp sea salt
- two tsps fresh sage
- two tbsps coconut oil

Directions:

1. Stir in the entire components, excluding the oil, inside a blending container. Refrigerate overnight, or for thirty mins.
2. Pour the oil into the solution. Form the solution into four patties.
3. Inside a lightly greased griddle placed at middling temp., cook the patties for five mins on all sides, or till their middle portions are no longer pink. You can also cook them by baking in the oven for twenty-five mins at 400F.

Per serving: Calories: 284kcal; Protein: 14g; Carbs: 36.9g; Fat: 9.4g

– Anti-Inflammatory Cookbook

7. Buckwheat Waffles

Preparation time: fifteen mins
Cooking time: six mins
Servings: two
Ingredients:

- half teacup of brown rice flour
- half tsp of baking soda
- one egg
- one teacup of buckwheat flour
- one tsp of baking powder
- half tsp of salt
- one tbsp of maple syrup
- half teacup of water
- one teacup of almond milk
- Coconut oil for the waffle iron
- one tsp of vanilla extract

Directions:

1. Whisk collectively the buckwheat flour, baking powder, rice flour, baking soda, and salt in a medium mixing dish.
2. Include the maple syrup, egg, and vanilla to the dry components. Whisk in the water and almond milk in a slow, steady stream till smooth.
3. The batter is absolutely free of lumps.
4. Allow ten mins for the batter to thicken slightly.
5. When the buckwheat is resting, it can settle to the bottom of the dish, so stir thoroughly before using.
6. Garnish the waffle iron with coconut oil and heat it.
7. In the waffle iron, pour the batter and cook as per to the manufacturer's guidelines.

Per serving: Calories: 282kcal; Protein: 9g; Carbs: 55g; Fat: 4g

8. Smoked Salmon Scrambled Eggs

Preparation time: five mins
Cooking time: eight mins
Servings: two
Ingredients:

- 3 ounces of flaked smoked salmon
- half tsp of freshly ground black pepper
- three-quarter tbsp of extra-virgin olive oil
- 4 beaten eggs

Directions:

1. Warm the olive oil in a griddle or pan at medium-high temp. till it starts shimmering.
2. Cook for around three mins, blending irregularly.
3. Set the eggs and pepper collectively inside a standard blending teacup. Include them to the griddle or pot and cook, stirring gently, for almost five mins, or till cooked.

Per serving: Calories: 236kcal; Protein: 19g; Carbs: 1g; Fat: 18g

9. Cucumber Bites

Preparation time: fifteen mins
Cooking time: zero mins
Servings: four
Ingredients:

- half teacup prepared hummus
- two tsps nutritional yeast
- ¼-½ teaspoon ground turmeric
- Pinch of red pepper cayenne
- Pinch of salt
- 1 cucumber, cut diagonally into ¼-½-inch thick slices
- one tsp black sesame seeds
- Fresh mint leaves, for garnishing

Directions:

1. Inside a container, mix collectively hummus, turmeric, cayenne and salt.
2. Transfer the hummus solution in the pastry bag and spread on each cucumber slice.
3. Serve while using garnishing of sesame seeds and mint leaves.

Per serving: Calories: 203kcal; Protein: 8g; Carbs: 20g; Fat: 4g

10. Yogurt, Berry, and Walnut Parfait

Preparation time: ten mins
Cooking time: zero mins
Servings: 2
Ingredients:

- two tbsps of honey
- two teacups of plain unsweetened coconut yogurt or plain unsweetened yogurt or almond yogurt
- one teacup of fresh blueberries
- half teacup of walnut pieces
- one teacup of fresh raspberries

Directions:

1. Stir the yogurt and honey together. Split into two bowls.
2. Sprinkle in blueberries and raspberries along with A quarter cup of chopped walnuts.

Per serving: Calories: 505kcal; Protein: 23g; Carbs: 56g; Fat: 22g

11. Spiced Popcorn

Preparation time: five mins
Cooking time: two mins
Servings: two-three
Ingredients:

- three tbsps coconut oil
- half teacup popping corn
- one tbsp olive oil
- one tsp ground turmeric
- quarter tsp garlic powder
- Salt, as required

Directions:

1. Inside a pan, dissolve coconut oil on medium-high temp.
2. Include popping corn and cover the pan tightly.
3. Cook, shaking the pan occasionally for almost one-two mins or till corn kernels begin to pop.
4. Take out from fire and transfer right into a big heatproof container.
5. Include essential olive oil and spices and mix thoroughly.
6. Serve instantly.

Per serving: Calories: 200kcal; Protein: 6g; Carbs: 12g; Fat: 4g

12. Poached Eggs

Preparation time: ten mins
Cooking time: forty mins
Servings: four
Ingredients:

- 3 tomatoes; chopped.
- 3 garlic cloves; crushed
- one tbsp ghee quarter tsp chili powder
- one tbsp cilantro; severed, 6 eggs
- 1 white onion; severed
- one red bell pepper; severed
- one tsp paprika
- one tsp cumin
- 1 serrano pepper; severed
- Salt and black pepper as required

Directions:

1. Warm up a pot with the ghee at middling temp.; include onion; stir and cook for ten mins.
2. Include Serrano pepper and garlic; stir and cook for one min.
3. Include red bell pepper; stir and cook for ten mins.
4. Include tomatoes, salt, pepper, chili powder, cumin and paprika; stir and cook for ten mins.
5. Crack eggs into the pot, flavour them with salt and pepper, cover pan then cook for six mins more.
6. Sprinkle cilantro at the end and serve.

Per serving: Calories: 300kcal; Protein: 14g; Carbs: 22gm; Fat: 12g

13. Plum, Pear and Berry-Baked Brown Rice

Preparation time: twelve mins
Cooking time: thirty mins
Servings: 2
Ingredients:

- one teacup water
- half teacup brown rice
- A pinch of cinnamon
- half tsp pure vanilla extract
- two tbsps pure maple syrup (divided)
- Sliced fruits: berries, pears, or plums
- A tweak of salt (optional)

Directions:

1. Warm up your oven at 400F.
2. Raise the water and brown rice solution to a boil in a pot placed at medium-high temp.. Stir in the cinnamon and vanilla extract. Decrease the temp. to medium-low. Simmer for eighteen mins, or till the brown rice is soft.
3. Fill two oven-safe bowls with equal portions of the rice. Pour a tablespoon of maple syrup into each bowl. Top the bowls with the sliced fruits and sprinkle over a tweak of salt.
4. Put the containers in the oven. Bake for twelve mins, or till the fruits start caramelizing and the syrup begins bubbling.

Per serving: Calories: 227kcal; Protein: 14g; Carbs: 32g; Fat: 6.3g

14. Spiced Morning Chia Pudding

Preparation time: ten mins
Cooking time: five mins
Servings: 1
Ingredients:

- half tsp. cinnamon
- one and half teacups cashew milk
- one-eighth tsp cardamom, grounded
- one-third teacup chia seeds
- one-eighth tsp cloves, grounded
- two tbsps maple syrup
- one tsp turmeric

Directions:

1. To begin with, blend the entire components inside a moderate container till thoroughly mixed.
2. Next, spoon the solution into a container and allow it to sit overnight.
3. In the morning, transfer to a cup and serve with toppings of your choice.

Per serving: Calories: 237kcal; Protein: 8.1g; Carbs: 28.9g; Fat: 8.1g

15. Overnight Muesli

Preparation time: ten mins

Cooking time: zero mins

Servings: two

Ingredients:

- one teacup of gluten-free rolled oats
- one teacup of coconut milk
- quarter teacup of no-includeed-sugar apple juice
- one tbsp of apple cider vinegar
- half cored and severed apple
- Dash ground cinnamon

Directions:

1. Blend the oats, apple juice, coconut milk, and vinegar inside a standard mixing dish.
2. Refrigerate overnight, covered.
3. The following day, include the sliced apple and a tweak of cinnamon to the muesli.

Per serving: Calories: 213kcal; Protein: 6g; Carbs: 39g; Fat: 4g

16. Gingerbread Oatmeal

Preparation time: ten mins

Cooking time: thirty mins

Servings: four

Ingredients:

- quarter tsp cardamom, grounded
- four teacups water
- quarter tsp allspice
- one teacup steel cut oats
- one-eighth tsp nutmeg
- one and half tbsps cinnamon, grounded
- quarter tsp ginger, grounded
- quarter tsp coriander, grounded
- Maple syrup, if desired
- quarter tsp cloves

Directions:

1. First, place the entire components inside a big saucepot at medium-high temp. and stir well.
2. Next, cook them for 6 to seven mins or till cooked.
3. Once finished, include the maple syrup.
4. Top it with dried fruits of your choice if desired.
5. Serve it hot or cold.
6. Tip: Avoid those spices which you don't prefer.

Per serving: Calories: 175kcal; Protein: 6g; Carbs: 32g; Fat: 32g

17. Spinach Fritters

Preparation time: fifteen mins
Cooking time: five mins
Servings: two-three
Ingredients:

- two teacups chickpea flour
- three-quarter tsp white sesame seeds
- half tsp garam masala powder
- half tsp red chili powder
- quarter tsp ground cumin
- 2 tweaks of baking soda
- Salt, as required
- one teacup water
- 12-14 fresh spinach leaves
- Olive oil, for frying

Directions:

1. Inside a big container, include the entire components excluding spinach and oil and mix till an easy solution forms.
2. Inside a sizable griddle, heat oil on middling temp.
3. Dip each spinach leaf in chickpea flour solution evenly and place in the hot oil in batches.
4. Cook, flipping occasionally for almost three to five mins or till golden brown from all sides.
5. Transfer the fritters onto paper towel lined plate.

Per serving: Calories: 211kcal; Protein: 9g; Carbs: 13g; Fat: 2g

18. Mushroom and Bell Pepper Omelet

Preparation time: ten mins
Cooking time: ten mins
Servings: 2
Ingredients:

- one sliced red bell pepper
- 6 beaten eggs
- one-eighth tsp ground black pepper
- two tbsps of extra virgin olive oil
- one teacup of sliced mushrooms
- half tsp of sea salt

Directions:

1. Warmth the olive oil in a broad non-stick pan at middling temp. till it shimmers.
2. Blend the mushrooms and red bell pepper in a mixing dish. Cook, blending continuously, for almost four mins, or till soft.
3. Whisk collectively the salt, eggs, and pepper inside a standard blending teacup. Set the eggs over the vegetables and cook for almost three mins, or till the edges of the eggs start to get established.
4. Gently raise the eggs away from the pan's sides with a rubber spatula. Let the uncooked egg to flow to the pan's edges by tilting it. Cook for two-five mins till the edges and core of the eggs are set.
5. Set the omelet in half with a spatula. To eat, break into wedges.

Per serving: Calories: 336kcal; Protein: 18g; Carbs: 7g; Fat: 27g

19. Warm Chia-Berry Non-dairy Yogurt

Preparation time: ten mins
Cooking time: five mins
Servings: two
Ingredients:

- one tbsp of maple syrup
- half vanilla bean halved lengthwise
- two teacups of unsweetened almond yogurt or coconut yogurt
- one (ten oz.) package frozen mixed berries, thawed
- one tbsp of freshly squeezed lemon juice
- half tbsp of chia seeds

Directions:

1. Blend the berries, lemon juice, maple syrup, and vanilla bean in a medium saucepan in a medium-high flame.
2. Get the solution to a boil, continuously stirring. Decrease the temp. to low heat then continue to cook for three mins.
3. Switch off the heat from the pan. Detach the vanilla bean from the solution and discard it. Include the chia seeds and mix thoroughly. Allow five to ten mins for the seeds to thicken.
4. Cover each bowl with one cup of yogurt and divide the fruit solution among both of them.

Per serving: Calories: 246kcal; Protein: 5g; Carbs: 35g; Fat: 10g

20. Chia Breakfast Pudding

Preparation time: ten mins
Cooking time: twenty-five mins
Servings: 2
Ingredients:

- half teacup of chia seeds
- half tsp of vanilla extract
- half teacup of frozen no-includeed-sugar pitted cherries, thawed, juice reserved, split
- half teacup of severed cashews, split
- one teacup of almond milk
- quarter teacup of maple syrup or honey

Directions:

1. Blend the chia seeds, almond milk, maple syrup, and vanilla in a quart container with a tight-fitting seal. Set aside after thoroughly shaking.
2. Pour the pudding into two containers and finish with a quarter cup of cherries and two tablespoons of cashews in each.

Per serving: Calories: 272kcal; Protein: 7g; Carbs: 38g; Fat: 14g

21. Coconut Pancakes

Preparation time: ten mins
Cooking time: five mins
Servings: two
Ingredients:

- half teacup of coconut, plus additional as needed
- half tbsp of maple syrup
- quarter teacup of coconut flour
- half tsp of salt
- 2 eggs
- half tbsp of coconut oil or almond butter
- half tsp of vanilla extract
- half tsp of baking soda

Directions:

1. Using an electric mixer, blend the coconut milk, maple syrup, eggs, coconut oil, and vanilla inside a standard blending teacup.
2. Blend the baking soda, coconut flour, and salt in a shallow blending container. Put the dry components with the wet components inside a blending container and beat 'til smooth and lump-free.
3. If the batter is too dense, include more liquid to fine it down to a typical pancake batter consistency.
4. Using coconut oil, lightly grease a big griddle or pan. Warm up the oven to medium-high.
5. Cook till golden brown on the rim. Cook for another two mins.
6. Continue to cook the leftover batter while stacking the pancake on a tray.

Per serving: Calories: 193kcal; Protein: 9g; Carbs: 15g; Fat: 11g

Chapter 3. Soups and Salads Recipes

22. Golden Mushroom Soup 30
23. Lime Spinach and Chickpeas Salad 30
24. Brown Rice and Chicken Soup 31
25. Lentils and Turmeric Soup 31
26. Garbanzo and Kidney Bean Salad 32
27. Avocado Side Salad 32
28. Coconut Cashew Soup with Butternut Squash 33
29. Beef & Vegetable Soup 33
30. Persimmon Salad 34
31. Italian Wedding Soup 34
32. Spicy Pumpkin Soup 35
33. Stuffed Pepper Soup 35
34. Wheatberry Salad 36
35. Orange Soup 36
36. Chipotle Squash Soup 37
37. Southwestern Bean-And-Pepper Salad 37
38. Chicken Noodle Soup 38
39. Roasted Carrot Soup 38
40. Chopped Tuna Salad 39
41. Chicken Squash Soup 39
42. Fennel Pear Soup 40
43. Nutty and Fruity Garden Salad 40
44. Couscous Salad 41
45. Shoepeg Corn Salad 41

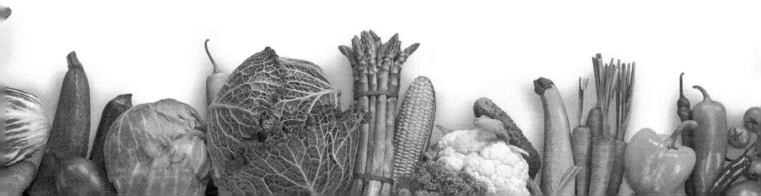

22. Golden Mushroom Soup

Preparation time: fifteen mins
Cooking time: 8 hours
Servings: six
Ingredients:

- one onion, finely severed
- one carrot, peeled and finely severed
- one fennel bulb, finely severed
- 1-pound fresh mushrooms, quartered
- 8 cups vegetable broth, poultry broth, or store-bought
- quarter teacup dry sherry
- one tsp dried thyme
- one tsp garlic powder
- half tsp of sea salt
- one-eighth tsp freshly ground black pepper

Directions:

1. In your slow cooker, blend the entire components, mixing to blend. Cover and set on low. Cook for eight hrs.

Per serving: Calories: 71kcal; Protein: 3g; Carbs: 15g; Fat: 0g

23. Lime Spinach and Chickpeas Salad

Preparation time: ten mins
Cooking time: zero mins
Servings: four
Ingredients:

- sixteen oz. tinned chickpeas, drained and washed
- two teacups baby spinach leaves
- half tbsp lime juice
- two tbsps olive oil
- one tsp cumin, ground
- A tweak of sea salt and black pepper
- half tsp chili flakes

Directions:

1. Inside a container, mix the chickpeas with the spinach and the remaining components, toss and serve cold.

Per serving: Calories: 240kcal; Protein: 12g; Carbs: 11.6g; Fat: 8.2g

24. Brown Rice and Chicken Soup

Preparation time: fifteen mins
Cooking time: four hrs
Servings: four
Ingredients:

- one-third teacups brown rice
- one severed leek
- one carved celery rib
- one and half teacups water
- half tsp kosher salt
- half bay leaf
- one-eighth tsp thyme (dried)
- quarter tsp black pepper (ground)
- one tbsp severed parsley
- half quart chicken broth (low sodium)
- one carved carrot
- three-quarter lb. of chicken thighs (skin and boneless)

Directions:

1. Bring half a teaspoon of salt and one teacup of water to a boil in a saucepot. To this, include the rice. Prepare over a fire that is moderate for thirty mins. The chicken pieces were browned in the oil. Once the chicken is done cooking, place it on a dish.
2. Using the similar skillet, cook the vegetables over medium heat for about three mins. Put the chicken pieces into the slow cooker at this point. Mix in some water and some broth. Cook for three hrs on the "low" setting. Place the other ingredients, saving the rice until last. Continue to cook for another ten minutes on "high." Upon removing the bay leaf, the dish should be served in containers.

Per serving: Calories: 208kcal; Protein: 2g; Carbs: 18g; Fat: 1g

25. Lentils and Turmeric Soup

Preparation time: ten mins
Cooking time: twenty-five mins
Servings: 3
Ingredients:

- two teacups of boiled lentils
- 2 carrots
- 1 shallot
- one tbsp of turmeric
- one teacup unsweetened almond milk
- one teacup low sodium vegetable broth
- one piece of garlic
- one tsp of parsley
- half teacup unsweetened soy yogurt
- 1 tweak of salt
- two tbsps of ghee
- 1 tweak of salt
- one tweak of cayenne pepper
- one tbsp of sesame seeds

Directions:

1. Wash and cut the carrots into pieces.
2. Chop the shallot. Chop the garlic together with the parsley.
3. Put the ghee in a saucepan and sauté the garlic and parsley for one min.
4. Include the lentils, carrots and sauté for five mins.
5. Include the cup of almond milk and the cup of broth, turmeric, salt and pepper and shallot.
6. Cook at moderate temp. for twenty-five mins.
7. Serve with the sesame seeds.

Per serving: Calories: 249kcal; Protein: 16g; Carbs: 41g; Fat: 4g

26. Garbanzo and Kidney Bean Salad

Preparation time: ten mins
Cooking time: zero mins
Servings: four
Ingredients:

- one (fifteen oz.) tin kidney beans, drained
- one (fifteen and half oz.) tin garbanzo beans, drained
- 1 lemon, zested and juiced
- one medium tomato, severed
- one tsp capers, washed and drained
- half teacup severed fresh parsley
- half tsp salt, or as required
- quarter teacup severed red onion
- three tbsps extra virgin olive oil

Directions:

1. Inside a salad container, whisk well lemon juice, olive oil and salt till dissolved.
2. Stir in garbanzo, kidney beans, tomato, red onion, parsley, and capers. Toss well to coat.
3. Allow flavors to mix for thirty mins by setting in the fridge.
4. Mix again prior to serving.

Per serving: Calories: 329kcal; Protein: 12.1g; Carbs: 46.6g; Fat: 12.0g

27. Avocado Side Salad

Preparation time: ten mins
Cooking time: zero mins
Servings: four
Ingredients:

- 4 blood oranges, slice into segments
- two tbsps olive oil
- A tweak of red pepper, crushed
- two avocados, peeled, cut into wedges
- 1 and half teacups baby arugula
- one tbsp lemon juice

Directions:

1. Mix the oranges with the oil, red pepper, avocados, arugula, almonds, and lemon juice in a bowl, then serve.

Per serving: Calories: 146kcal; Protein: 15g; Carbs: 8g; Fat: 7g

28. Coconut Cashew Soup with Butternut Squash

Preparation time: ten mins
Cooking time: twenty mins
Servings: six
Ingredients:

- two tbsps coconut oil
- three-quarter teacup toasted cashews
- two red chili peppers, sowed and cubed
- three garlic pieces, skinned and crushed
- one white onion, cubed
- one and half tbsps ginger, skinned and crushed
- two carrots, severed
- one small butternut squash, shared, cubed
- one small Napa cabbage, shredded
- two teacups green beans, clipped
- three teacups vegetable broth
- one (fourteen oz.) tin full-fat coconut milk
- half tsp salt
- Freshly ground black pepper
- one teacup mung bean sprouts
- four tbsps toasted coconut shavings

Directions:

1. Dissolve the coconut oil inside a large stockpot at a temp. setting of medium.
2. Include the cashews to the pan and cook them for two mins. Pull it out of the pot and put it to the side.
3. Sauté the peppers, garlic, and onion for a minimum of six mins after placing them in the pan. After that, add the ginger and carrots, and sauté them for a minimum of three mins, or till the carrots and squash start to become more pliable.
4. Combine the cabbage, green beans, broth, coconut milk, salt, and pepper, and then blend in the cabbage and green beans. Simmer for fifteen mins. Take out the pot from the flame.
5. Include the bean sprouts and the coconut shavings and stir to combine.
6. Ladle the soup into individual dishes, and serve at once.

Per serving: Calories: 340kcal; Protein: 7g; Carbs: 23g; Fat: 25g

29. Beef & Vegetable Soup

Preparation time: five mins
Cooking time: fifty-five mins
Servings: four
Ingredients:

- one lb. beef stew
- three and half teacups water
- one teacup raw sliced onions
- half teacup of frozen green peas
- one teaspoon black pepper
- half teacup frozen okra
- half tsp basil
- half teacup frozen carrots, cubed
- half tsp thyme
- half teacup of frozen corn

Directions:

1. Put a big pot at moderate temp., then include the beef, water, thyme, basil, and black pepper.
2. Cook the beef for forty-five mins on a simmer.
3. Stir in the okra and other vegetables and cook till the meat is al dente.
4. Serve warm.

Per serving: Calories: 163kcal; Protein: 8g; Carbs: 19.3g; Fat: 6.5g

30. Persimmon Salad

Preparation time: ten mins
Cooking time: zero mins
Servings: four
Ingredients:

- Seeds from one pomegranate
- two persimmons, cored and sliced
- five teacups baby arugula
- six tbsps green onions, severed
- 4 navel oranges, cut into segments
- quarter teacup white vinegar
- one-third teacup olive oil
- three tbsps pine nuts
- one and half tsps orange zest, grated
- two tbsps orange juice
- one tbsp coconut sugar
- ½ shallot, severed
- A tweak of cinnamon powder

Directions:

1. Inside a salad container, blend the pomegranate seeds with persimmons, arugula, green onions, and oranges and toss.
2. Inside a separate container, blend the vinegar with the oil, pine nuts, orange zest, orange juice, sugar, shallot, and cinnamon, whisk thoroughly, include to the salad, toss and serve as a side dish.

Per serving: Calories: 310kcal; Protein: 7g; Carbs: 33g; Fat: 16g

31. Italian Wedding Soup

Preparation time: fifteen mins
Cooking time: 7 hours
Servings: six
Ingredients:

- one lb. ground turkey breast
- one and half teacups cooked brown rice
- one onion, grated
- quarter teacup severed fresh parsley
- one egg, beaten
- one tsp garlic powder
- one tsp sea salt, split
- six teacups poultry broth or store-bought
- one-eighth tsp freshly ground black pepper
- Tweak of red pepper flakes
- one lb. kale, tough stems detached, leaves severed

Directions:

1. Put the turkey breast, rice, onion, parsley, egg, garlic powder, and a half tsp of salt into a small container and mix well. After forming the combination into meatballs with a diameter of 12 inches, place them in the slow cooker.
2. After that, include the broth, the extra black pepper, the remainder red pepper flakes, and the remainder of the half tsp of sea salt. Cook, covered, on low heat for seven to eight hrs. Prior to serving, incorporate the kale by stirring it in. Keep the lid on and continue to simmer till the kale has wilted.

Per serving: Calories: 302kcal; Protein: 29g; Carbs: 29g; Fat: 7g

32. Spicy Pumpkin Soup

Preparation time: ten mins
Cooking time: forty-five mins
Servings: 5
Ingredients:

- two teacups of lentils
- two teacups of squash
- two tomatoes
- three teacups low sodium vegetable broth
- two red onions
- 6 leaves of dill
- 6 basil leaves
- 1 tweak of salt
- two tbsps of olive oil
- one tweak of salt
- one tweak of cayenne pepper
- one chili
- two pieces of garlic

Directions:

1. Cut the tomato into cubes, chop the onion with the chili. Inside a saucepot, fry the onion and include the tomato, cook for five mins.
2. Include the broth, lentils, salt, pepper and garlic, cook for forty mins.
3. Coarsely chop the dill and basil leaves, include them to the soup and cook for the last five mins.
4. The soup can be eaten like this or pureed.

Per serving: Calories: 133kcal; Protein: 6g; Carbs: 17g; Fat: 6g

33. Stuffed Pepper Soup

Preparation time: fifteen mins
Cooking time: eight hrs & ten mins
Servings: 6
Ingredients:

- one lb. ground beef (drained)
- one severed onion (large)
- two teacups tomatoes (cubed)
- 2 severed green peppers
- two teacups tomato sauce
- 1 tbs. beef bouillon
- three teacups of water
- Pepper
- one tsp of salt
- one teacup of cooked rice (white)

Directions:

1. Place the entire components inside a cooker. Cook for eight hrs on "low." Serve hot.

Per serving: Calories: 216.1kcal; Protein: 18.3g; Carbs: 21.8g; Fat: 5.2g

34. Wheatberry Salad

Preparation time: ten mins
Cooking time: fifty mins
Servings: two
Ingredients:

- quarter teacup of wheat berries
- one teacup of water
- one tsp salt
- two tbsps walnuts, severed
- one tbsp chives, severed
- quarter teacup fresh parsley, severed
- two oz. pomegranate seeds
- one tbsp canola oil
- one tsp chili flakes

Directions:
1. Inside a saucepan, combine the wheat berries with the water.
2. Sprinkle the components with salt and continue to cook them at a low simmer for fifty mins.
3. In the meantime, combine chopped walnuts, chives, parsley, pomegranate seeds, and red pepper flakes in a mixing container.
4. Once the wheatberry has finished cooking, place it in the container with the walnut solution.
5. Pour in the canola oil and thoroughly toss the salad.

Per serving: Calories: 160kcal; Protein: 3.4g; Carbs: 12g; Fat: 11.8g

35. Orange Soup

Preparation time: twelve mins
Cooking time: forty-five mins
Servings: four
Ingredients:

- two teacups of carrots
- two teacups of squash
- 2 sweet potatoes
- 1 grated ginger root
- two teacups of low sodium vegetable broth
- one teacup unsweetened coconut milk
- one tsp of paprika
- 7 basil leaves
- 1 tweak of salt
- two tbsps of olive oil
- one tweak of salt
- one tweak of cayenne pepper

Directions:
1. Chop the basil leaves and put them in a pan with the oil and paprika.
2. Dice the sweet potatoes, pumpkin and carrots and sauté for five mins, mixing with a spoon.
3. Include the broth and coconut milk, include the salt, pepper and ginger.
4. Boil for forty-five mins over moderate heat. Serve warm.

Per serving: Calories: 155kcal; Protein: 3g; Carbs: 20gm; Fat: 8g

36. Chipotle Squash Soup

Preparation time: fifteen mins
Cooking time: four hrs & twenty mins
Servings: 6
Ingredients:

- six teacups butternut squash (cubed)
- half teacup severed onion
- two tsps adobo chipotle
- two teacups chicken broth
- one tbsp brown sugar
- quarter teacup tart apple (severed)
- one teacup yogurt (Greek style)
- two tbsps chives (severed)

Directions:

1. Put the remaining components in the slow cooker, with the exception of the yogurt, the chives, and the apple. Cook for four hrs on the "low" setting. Next, place all of the cooked components inside a high-powered mixer or blending container and purée them. The puree should now be placed in the slow cooker.
2. Cook on "Low" for a further twenty mins after adding the yogurt. Apples and chives should be used as a garnish. To serve hot, use containers that have been warmed.

Per serving: Calories: 102kcal; Protein: 2g; Carbs: 22g; Fat: 1g

37. Southwestern Bean-And-Pepper Salad

Preparation time: six mins
Cooking time: zero mins
Servings: four
Ingredients:

- one tin pinto beans, drained
- two bell peppers, cored and severed
- one teacup corn kernels
- Salt
- Freshly ground black pepper
- Juice of two limes
- one tbsp olive oil
- one avocado, severed

Directions:

1. Inside a big container, combine the beans, peppers, corn, salt, and pepper. Blend well.
2. Squeeze some fresh lime juice into some olive oil, and then mix the two together. Over the next half an hour, place the salad in the refrigerator to chill. Include avocado instantly prior to serving.

Per serving: Calories: 245kcal; Protein: 8g; Carbs: 32g; Fat: 11g

38. Chicken Noodle Soup

Preparation time: ten mins.
Cooking time: twenty-five mins.
Servings: four
Ingredients:

- quarter teacup extra-virgin olive oil
- three celery stalks, cut into quarter-inch slices
- 2 medium carrots, cut into quarter inch dice
- one small onion, cut into quarter inch dice
- one fresh rosemary sprig
- four teacups chicken broth
- 8 ounces gluten-free penne
- one tsp salt
- quarter tsp black pepper, freshly ground
- two teacups cubed rotisserie chicken
- quarter teacup severed fresh flat-leaf parsley

Directions:
1. Inside a suitable pot, warm the oil over high temp.
2. Include the celery, carrots, onion, and rosemary and sauté till softened, five-seven mins.
3. Include the broth, penne, salt, and pepper and bring to a boil.
4. Decrease its temp. to a simmer and cook till the penne is soft, eight-ten mins.
5. Take out and discard the rosemary sprig, and include the chicken and parsley.
6. Decrease its temp. to low. Cook till the chicken is warmed through, almost five mins, and serve.

Per serving: Calories: 302kcal; Protein: 24g; Carbs: 19.2g; Fat: 14.7g

39. Roasted Carrot Soup

Preparation time: fifteen mins
Cooking time: fifty mins
Servings: 4
Ingredients:

- eight big carrots, washed and skinned
- six tbsps olive oil
- one quart broth
- Cayenne pepper as required
- Sunflower seeds and pepper as required

Directions:
1. Warm up the oven to 425° F. Put carrots on a baking sheet, spray with olive oil, and roast in the oven for thirty to forty-five mins.
2. Place the roasted carrots inside a mixer with the broth, and purée the mixture. Transfer to a saucepot, then boil the soup.
3. Flavour with ground black pepper, cayenne pepper, and sunflower seeds. Spray olive oil. Serve, and have fun with it!

Per serving: Calories: 222kcal; Protein: 5g; Carbs: 7g; Fat: 18g

40. Chopped Tuna Salad

Preparation time: fifteen mins
Cooking time: zero mins
Servings: four
Ingredients:

- two tbsps extra-virgin olive oil
- two tbsps lemon juice
- two tsps Dijon mustard
- half tsp kosher salt
- quarter tsp freshly ground black pepper
- 12 olives, pitted and severed
- half teacup celery, cubed
- half teacup red onion, cubed
- half teacup red bell pepper, cubed
- half teacup fresh parsley, severed
- two (six oz.) tins no-salt-includeed tuna packed in water, drained
- six teacups baby spinach

Directions:

1. Mix the olive oil, lemon juice, mustard, salt, and black pepper inside a moderate container.
2. Include in the olives, celery, onion, bell pepper, and parsley and mix thoroughly. Include the tuna and gently incorporate.
3. Split the spinach evenly among 4 plates or containers. Spoon the tuna salad evenly on top of the spinach.

Per serving: Calories: 220kcal; Protein: 25g; Carbs: 7g; Fat: 11g

41. Chicken Squash Soup

Preparation time: fifteen mins
Cooking time: 5 hours & thirty mins
Servings: 3
Ingredients:

- half butternut squash (large)
- one piece garlic
- one and quarter quarts broth (vegetable or chicken)
- one-eighth tsp pepper (white)
- half tbsp severed parsley
- two crushed sage leaves
- one tbsp olive oil
- quarter severed onion (white)
- one-sixteenth tsp. black pepper (cracked)
- half tbsp of pepper flakes (chili)
- half tsp severed rosemary

Directions:

1. Warm up the oven to 400° Fahrenheit. Prepare a baking tray by greasing it. Cook the squash for thirty minutes in an oven that has been warmed up. Place it on a platter, and allow it to cool down there. In the oil, soften the onion and garlic until translucent.
2. Using a spoon, take out the meat from the baked squash and include it to the onion and garlic that has been sautéed. Mix everything up thoroughly. The slow cooker should have a half quart of the broth poured into it. Combine the squash in a separate container. Cook for four hours on the "low" setting. Create a silky purée by blending the ingredients inside a mixer.
3. Place the pureed ingredients into the slow cooker. Include the remaining portions of the broth as well as any additional components. Cook for an additional hour on the "high" setting. To serve, use containers of warm soup.

Per serving: Calories: 158kcal; Protein: 3g; Carbs: 24g; Fat: 3g

42. Fennel Pear Soup

Preparation time: ten mins
Cooking time: fifteen mins
Servings: four
Ingredients:

- two tbsps extra-virgin olive oil
- two leeks, white part only, sliced
- one fennel bulb, cut into quarter inch-thick slices
- two pears, skinned, cored, and cut into half inch cubes
- one tsp salt
- quarter tsp black pepper
- half teacup cashews
- three teacups water or vegetable broth
- two teacups spinach or arugula

Directions:

1. Warm the olive oil inside a Dutch oven that is appropriate for the task at a high temp.
2. Include the fennel and leeks to the pan. Sauté for five mins.
3. Include the pears, then season them with salt and pepper. Sauté for extra three mins.
4. Raise the soup to a boil, then include the water and cashews and stir to combine. Bring it to a simmer, then continue cooking it for another five mins while it is slightly closed.
5. Fold the spinach into the mixture.
6. Transfer the cooked soup to a mixer and, working in stages if required, purée the soup till it is completely even.

Per serving: Calories: 229kcal; Protein: 5.4g; Carbs: 26.2g; Fat: 12.6g

43. Nutty and Fruity Garden Salad

Preparation time: ten mins
Cooking time: zero mins
Servings: two
Ingredients:

- six teacups baby spinach
- half teacup severed walnuts, toasted
- one ripe red pear, sliced
- one ripe persimmon, sliced
- one tsp garlic crushed
- one shallot, crushed
- one tbsp extra-virgin olive oil
- two tbsps fresh lemon juice
- one tsp wholegrain mustard

Directions:

1. Inside a big salad container, combine and thoroughly blend the garlic, shallot, oil, lemon juice, and mustard.
2. Include the spinach, the persimmon, and the pear. Shake to ensure an even coating.
3. Before serving, sprinkle the dish with the severed pecans.

Per serving: Calories: 332kcal; Protein: 7g; Carbs: 37g; Fat: 21g

44. Couscous Salad

Preparation time: ten mins
Cooking time: six mins
Servings: four
Ingredients:

- one-third teacup couscous
- one-third teacup chicken stock
- quarter tsp ground black pepper
- three-quarter tsp ground coriander
- half tsp salt
- quarter tsp paprika
- quarter tsp turmeric
- one tbsp butter
- two oz. chickpeas, tinned, drained
- one teacup fresh arugula, severed
- two oz. sun-dried tomatoes, severed
- one oz. feta cheese, smashed
- one tbsp canola oil

Directions:

1. Raise the stock made from chicken to a boil.
2. Stir in the couscous, freshly ground black pepper, freshly ground coriander, paprika, and turmeric. Stir in the chickpeas and the butter. After giving the contents a good stir, cover it with the cover.
3. Set a timer for six mins and allow the couscous to immerse in the heated chicken stock.
4. In the meantime, blend the arugula, sun-dried tomatoes, and Feta cheese in the blending container.
5. Stir in the canola oil and the cooked couscous combination.
6. Give the salad a thorough toss.

Per serving: Calories: 18kcal; Protein: 6g; Carbs: 21.1g; Fat: 9g

45. Shoepeg Corn Salad

Preparation time: ten mins
Cooking time: zero mins
Servings: four
Ingredients:

- quarter teacup Greek yogurt
- one teacup shoepeg corn, drained
- half teacup cherry tomatoes shared
- one jalapeno pepper, severed
- one tbsp lemon juice
- three tbsps fresh cilantro, severed
- one tbsp chives, severed

Directions:

1. Inside the container with the salad ingredients, combine the corn on the cob, cherry tomatoes, jalapeño pepper, chives, and fresh cilantro.
2. Mix in some freshly squeezed lemon juice and Greek yogurt. Toss the salad thoroughly.
3. Put it inside the fridge, and you can keep it there for a maximum of one day.

Per serving: Calories: 49kcal; Protein: 2.7g; Carbs: 9.4g; Fat: 0.7g

Chapter 4. Main Course Recipes

MEAT-BASED RECIPES

46. Pork with Olives 43
47. Pork with Thyme Sweet Potatoes 43
48. Pork Kabobs with Bell Peppers 44
49. Mustard Pork Mix 44
50. Spiced Ground Beef 45
51. Beef with Carrot & Broccoli 46
52. Cranberry Pork 46
53. Crispy Beef Carnitas 47
54. Oregano Pork 48
55. Pork with Chili Zucchinis and Tomatoes 48

46. Pork with Olives

Preparation time: ten mins
Cooking time: forty mins
Servings: four
Ingredients:

- one yellow onion, severed
- four pork chops
- two tbsps olive oil
- one tbsp sweet paprika
- two tbsps balsamic vinegar
- quarter teacup kalamata olives, eroded and severed
- one tbsp cilantro, severed
- Tweak of of sea salt
- Tweak of black pepper

Directions:

1. Put the oil inside a skillet and bring it up to a middling temp. Include the onion and cook it for five mins.
2. After the beef has been browned for an additional five mins, include the vegetables.
3. Include the remaining components, give everything a good shake, and then continue to cook it at a heat setting of medium for around half an hour.

Per serving: Calories: 280kcal; Protein: 21g; Carbs: 10g; Fat: 11g

47. Pork with Thyme Sweet Potatoes

Preparation time: ten mins
Cooking time: thirty-five mins
Servings: four
Ingredients:

- two sweet potatoes, cut into wedges
- four pork chops
- three spring onions, severed
- one tbsp thyme, severed
- two tbsps olive oil
- four garlic pieces, crushed
- Tweak of of sea salt
- Tweak of black pepper
- half teacup vegetable stock
- half tbsp chives, severed

Directions:

1. Place the pork chops, potatoes, and the remaining components into a roasting pot. Give everything a little toss, then place in the oven and bake at 390 °Fahrenheit for thirty-five mins.
2. Place equal portions of each item on individual plates and serve.

Per serving: Calories: 210kcal; Protein: 10g; Carbs: 12g; Fat: 12.2g

48. Pork Kabobs with Bell Peppers

Preparation time: ten mins
Cooking time: twelve mins
Servings: four
Ingredients:

- two red bell peppers, severed
- two lbs. pork, cubed
- one red onion, severed
- one zucchini, sliced
- Juice of one lime
- two tbsps chili powder
- two tbsps hot sauce
- half tbsps cumin powder
- quarter teacup olive oil
- quarter teacup salsa
- Tweak of of sea salt
- Tweak of of black pepper

Directions:

1. Put the salsa, lime juice, oil, hot sauce, chili powder, cumin, salt, and black pepper into a container and whisk all of the ingredients together.
2. Thread the meat, bell peppers, zucchini, and onion onto skewers, and then smear them with salsa prior to serving.
3. Put them on a grill that has been prepared to a temperature of medium-high, and cook them for six minutes total on both ends.
4. Split across plates and serve.
5. Relish!

Per serving: Calories: 300kcal; Protein: 14g; Carbs: 12g; Fat: 5g

49. Mustard Pork Mix

Preparation time: ten mins
Cooking time: thirty-five mins
Servings: four
Ingredients:

- two shallots, severed
- one lb. pork stew meat, cubed
- two garlic pieces, crushed
- two tbsps olive oil
- quarter teacup Dijon mustard
- two tbsps chives, severed
- one tsp cumin, ground
- one tsp rosemary, dried
- Tweak of of sea salt
- Tweak of black pepper

Directions:

1. Bring a frying pot with the oil to a medium-high temp., include the shallots, and cook them for five mins while mixing often.
2. Place the meat in the pan and continue to brown it for another five mins.
3. Include the other components, give everything a good stir, and continue cooking over middling temp. for another twenty-five mins.
4. Distribute the mixture evenly among the dishes, and serve.

Per serving: Calories: 280kcal; Protein: 17g; Carbs: 11.8g; Fat: 14.3g

50. Spiced Ground Beef

Preparation time: ten mins
Cooking time: twenty-two mins
Servings: five
Ingredients:

- two tbsps coconut oil
- two whole cloves
- two whole cardamoms
- one (two-inch piece cinnamon stick
- two bay leaves
- one tsp cumin seeds
- two onions, severed
- Salt, as required
- half tbsp garlic paste
- half tbsp fresh ginger paste
- one lb. lean ground beef
- one and half tsps fennel seeds powder
- one tsp ground cumin
- one and half tsps red chili powder
- one-eighth tsp ground turmeric
- Freshly ground black pepper, as required
- one teacup coconut milk
- quarter teacup water
- quarter teacup fresh cilantro, severed

Directions:

1. Bring the oil to a simmer inside a big griddle over middling temp.
2. After around twenty to a couple of secs of sautéing, incorporate the cloves, cardamoms, cinnamon stick, bay leaves, and cumin seeds.
3. After the onion has been sautéed for around three to four mins, include two pinches of salt.
4. After approximately two mins of sautéing, include the garlic-ginger paste.
5. After approximately four to five mins of cooking, include the meat and break it up with a spoon while it's cooking.
6. Keep the lid on and continue cooking for about five mins.
7. While continuing to stir, include the spices, and continue cooking for extra two to two and a half mins.
8. After mixing in the coconut milk and the water, continue to cook for another seven to eight mins.
9. Flavour with salt and remove from the fire instantly.
10. Serve the dish hot with the cilantro on top as a garnish.

Per serving: Calories: 444kcal; Protein: 39g; Carbs: 29g; Fat: 15g

51. Beef with Carrot & Broccoli

Preparation time: fifteen mins
Cooking time: fourteen mins
Servings: four
Ingredients:

- two tbsps coconut oil, split
- two medium garlic pieces, crushed
- one lb. beef sirloin steak, sliced into fine strips
- Salt, as required
- quarter teacup chicken broth
- two tsps fresh ginger, grated
- one tbsp ground flax seeds
- half tsp red pepper flakes, crushed
- quarter tsp freshly ground black pepper
- one big carrot, skinned and cut finely
- two teacups broccoli florets
- one medium scallion, cut finely

Directions:

1. Put one tbsp of oil into a griddle and warm it over medium-high temp.
2. Put garlic and sauté almost one min.
3. Include the ground beef along with the salt, and continue to cook for almost four-five mins, or until the steak has browned.
4. Place the meat inside a container by using a slotted spoon to do the transfer.
5. Take out any liquid that may have accumulated in the pan.
6. In a dish, combine the broth, the ginger, the flax seeds, the crushed red pepper, and the ground black pepper, then stir well.
7. Put the residual oil in the griddle and warm it over medium-low temp.
8. Put the carrot, broccoli, and ginger mixture into the pan, and then heat for almost three to four mins, or until the vegetables are cooked to the appropriate degree.
9. Combine the beef and scallion, and then proceed to cook for approximately three to four mins.

Per serving: Calories: 412kcal; Protein: 35g; Carbs: 28g; Fat: 13g

52. Cranberry Pork

Preparation time: ten mins
Cooking time: eight hrs
Servings: four
Ingredients:

- one and half lbs. pork roast
- half tsp fresh grated ginger
- one tbsp coconut flour
- A tweak of mustard powder
- A tweak of salt and black pepper
- half teacup cranberries
- quarter teacup water
- Juice of half lemon
- two garlic pieces, crushed

Directions:

1. Place the roast in the slow cooker and combine it with the ginger, flour, mustard, salt, pepper, cranberries, water, lemon juice, and garlic. Stir until well combined. Cook, covered, on the lowest possible heat setting for a minimum of eight hrs. Cut all into bite-sized pieces, then distribute it evenly among the dishes, and serve.
2. Relish!

Per serving: Calories: 261kcal; Protein: 17g; Carbs: 9g; Fat: 4g

53. Crispy Beef Carnitas

Preparation time: twenty mins
Cooking time: twenty mins
Servings: eight
Ingredients:

- four slices turkey, cubed
- four pieces garlic, crushed
- one big onion, cubed
- three-four lbs. chuck shoulder roast
- one tbsp fine Himalayan salt
- two tsps ground black pepper
- two tsps oregano, dried
- two tsps ground cumin
- three tbsps coconut oil
- one teacup bone broth
- Juice of three limes
- quarter teacup coconut aminos
- two bay leaves

FOR SERVING:

- six street taco tortillas, warm
- fiesta guacamole
- red onions, pickled

Directions:

1. Inside a big pan, warm the turkey, garlic, and onions in the griddle at medium-high temp. for almost five mins, till the turkey is nicely browned. Take out the solution from the griddle and place it in a slow cooker.
2. While the turkey combination is cooking, slice the roast into two parts of similar size and put them flat on a cutting board. Rub the entire solution onto the roast, and then transfer any remaining seasonings from the cutting board to the slow cooker. The salt, pepper, oregano, and cumin should be combined inside a container, and then rubbed together.
3. Dissolve the coconut oil in the frying pan and sear the meat for two mins on all sides. After the meat has been browned, place it in the slow cooker, then pour the broth into the griddle to deglaze it. Finally, use a scraper to remove any remaining meat and seasonings. The tasty pieces should be lifted from the griddle, and the stock should be poured into the slow cooker.
4. Include the lime juice and coconut aminos to the slow cooker, and then turn the beef several times in the turkey-onion combination that is in the slow cooker.
5. Organize the bay leaves in a decorative pattern on top of the meat, then cover the slow cooker with the cover. Prepare over a low temp. for around ten hrs.
6. Take out the meat from the slow cooker and place it on a sheet pot. Using two forks, shred the beef that has been cooked in the slow cooker. Place the beef under the broiler for about eight mins, or till it reaches the desired level of crispiness, and then pour two ladlefuls of the liquid from the slow cooker over it.
7. To make the perfect taco, place a mound of carnitas in the center of a tortilla, dollop some guacamole on top, and sprinkle some pickled onions on top.
8. Place any leftovers in a sealed container and store them in the refrigerator for almost five days; to reheat, sauté them in a griddle at middling temp.

Per serving: Calories: 213kcal; Protein: 23.2g; Carbs: 5.6g; Fat: 11g

54. Oregano Pork

Preparation time: ten mins
Cooking time: eight hrs
Servings: four
Ingredients:

- two lbs. pork roast, sliced
- two tbsps oregano, severed
- quarter teacup balsamic vinegar
- one teacup tomato paste
- one tbsp sweet paprika
- one tsp onion powder
- two tbsps chili powder
- two garlic pieces, crushed
- A tweak of salt and black pepper

Directions:

1. Place the roast, the oregano, the vinegar, and the remaining components into your slow cooker. Give everything a good stir, then cover and simmer on Low heat for eight hrs.
2. Place equal portions of each item on individual plates and serve.

Per serving: Calories: 300kcal; Protein: 24g; Carbs: 12g; Fat: 5g

55. Pork with Chili Zucchinis and Tomatoes

Preparation time: ten mins
Cooking time: thirty-five mins
Servings: 4
Ingredients:

- two tomatoes, cubed
- two lbs. pork stew meat, cubed
- four scallions, severed
- two tbsps olive oil
- one zucchini, sliced
- Juice of one lime
- two tbsps chili powder
- half tbsps cumin powder
- Tweak of of sea salt
- Tweak of black pepper

Directions:

1. Place the oil in a skillet and bring it up to a midddling temp. Include the scallions and cook them for five mins.
2. Include the meat and continue to brown it for another five mins.
3. Include the tomatoes as well as the remaining components, combine, and continue to simmer at middling temp. for another twenty-five mins. After that, split the mixture among plates and serve.

Per serving: Calories: 300kcal; Protein: 14g; Carbs: 12g; Fat: 5g

POULTRY-BASED RECIPES

56. Chicken Lettuce Cups 50
57. Chicken with Coconut Milk 50
58. Easy Turkey Lettuce Wraps 51
59. Chicken with Snow Peas and Brown Rice 51
60. Orange Chicken Legs 52
61. Turkey Sausages 52
62. Rosemary Chicken 53
63. Cinnamon Chicken Pesto Pasta 53
64. Roasted Chicken 54

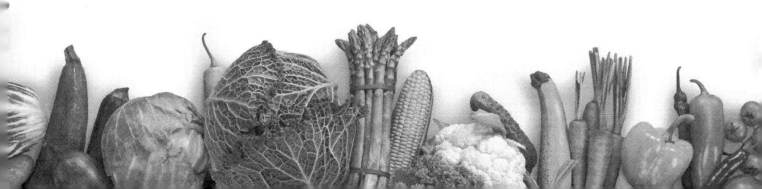

56. Chicken Lettuce Cups

Preparation time: twenty mins
Cooking time: ten mins
Servings: 4
Ingredients:

- one lb. grilled boneless skin-on chicken breast, cut into half inch cubes
- one teacup shredded carrots
- half teacup finely cut radishes
- two heads butter lettuce, 8 lettuce cups total
- 2 tbsps. severed fresh cilantro
- half teacup toasted sesame oil
- three tbsps freshly squeezed lime juice
- one tbsp coconut aminos
- one fine slice fresh ginger
- one garlic clove
- 2 scallions, sliced thin
- one tsp lime zest
- one tbsp sesame seeds, split

Directions:

1. Put the lettuce cups on a serving platter.
2. Split the scallions, chicken, radishes, carrots, and cilantro evenly between the lettuce cups.
3. Inside a blending container, blend the lime juice, ginger, sesame oil, garlic, coconut aminos, and lime zest. Blend till smooth.
4. Spray the chicken and vegetables with the dressing and spray with sesame seeds. Serve.

Per serving: Calories: 342kcal; Protein: 7g; Carbs: 13g; Fat: 30g

57. Chicken with Coconut Milk

Preparation time: ten mins
Cooking time: 6 hours
Servings: four-six
Ingredients:

- six bone-in skin-on chicken thighs
- two garlic pieces, smashed
- one tbsp coconut oil
- one onion, sliced
- two tsps curry powder
- one tsp salt
- quarter tsp freshly ground black pepper
- one (thirteen and half oz.) can unsweetened coconut milk
- three teacups chicken broth
- 2 scallions, sliced
- quarter teacup severed fresh cilantro

Directions:

1. Grease the slow cooker with the coconut oil.
2. Put in the garlic, chicken, salt, onion, curry powder, coconut milk, pepper, and chicken broth. Cover the slow cooker and cook for 6 hours on high.
3. Garnish with the cilantro and scallions. Serve.

Per serving: Calories: 652kcal; Protein: 32g; Carbs: 10g; Fat: 56g

58. Easy Turkey Lettuce Wraps

Preparation time: ten mins
Cooking time: twenty mins
Servings: four
Ingredients:

- one lb. ground turkey
- 8 small romaine lettuce leaves
- one small red onion, cubed
- 2 crushed garlic cloves
- two tbsps freshly squeezed lemon juice
- two tsps fish sauce
- 4 shallots, sliced
- two tbsps fresh parsley, crushed
- one tbsp fresh sage, crushed
- one tbsp maple syrup
- quarter tsp red pepper flakes

Directions:

1. Inside a big griddle, cook the turkey for ten mins at medium-high temp., tossing and breaking up the meat.
2. Place in the onion and garlic, then cook for almost ten mins, mixing, 'til the onions are soft and the meat is cooked.
3. Off the heat and remove griddle. Whisk in the shallots, sage, lemon juice, parsley, fish sauce, maple syrup, and red pepper flakes till well combined.
4. Pour the meat solution on each romaine leaf. Serve warm or cold.

Per serving: Calories: 143kcal; Protein: 24g; Carbs: 9g; Fat: 2g

59. Chicken with Snow Peas and Brown Rice

Preparation time: ten mins
Cooking time: five mins
Servings: four
Ingredients:

- two teacups cooked brown rice
- one tbsp coconut oil
- 2 scallions, sliced
- one teacup cooked chicken, cut into half inch cubes
- four oz. snow peas, strings taken out
- half teacup chicken broth
- one tsp salt
- half tsp ground ginger
- one tsp toasted sesame oil
- one tsp coconut aminos

Directions:

1. Inside a big pot, place it at high temp. and begin to dissolve the coconut oil. Rice and chicken should then be added. Sauté for around two mins.
2. Put in some salt, snow peas, some ginger, and some chicken broth. Conceal the pot, reduce the heat to low, and continue cooking the snow peas for three mins, or till they turn a vibrant green color.
3. Take the pot from the stove and set it aside. Stir in the scallions, sesame oil, and coconut aminos until well combined.

Per serving: Calories: 285kcal; Protein: 15g; Carbs: 39g; Fat: 7g

60. Orange Chicken Legs

Preparation time: ten mins
Cooking time: eight hrs
Servings: four
Ingredients:

- Zest of one orange
- Juice of one orange
- quarter teacup red vinegar
- A tweak of salt and black pepper
- four chicken legs
- five garlic pieces, crushed
- one red onion, cut into wedges
- seven oz. tinned peaches, shared
- half teacup severed parsley

Directions:

1. Combine the orange zest, orange juice, vinegar, salt, pepper, garlic, onion, peaches, and parsley inside a slow cooker. Blend in the orange juice first, then add the vinegar. After adding the chicken, give everything a good stir, then conceal and cook on Low for eight hrs. Split amongst plates and serve.
2. Relish!

Per serving: Calories: 251kcal; Protein: 8g; Carbs: 14g; Fat: 4g

61. Turkey Sausages

Preparation time: ten mins
Cooking time: ten mins
Servings: 2
Ingredients:

- quarter tsp salt
- one-eighth tsp garlic powder
- one-eighth tsp onion powder
- one tsp fennel seed
- one lb. 7%g; fat: ground turkey

Directions:

1. Press the fennel seed and put together turkey with fennel seed, garlic, onion powder, and salt in a small cup.
2. Cover the container and refrigerate overnight.
3. Prepare the turkey with flavouring into different portions with a circle form and press them into patties ready to be cooked.
4. Cook at middling temp. till browned.
5. Cook it for one to two minutes per side and serve them warm. Enjoy!

Per serving: Calories: 55kcal; Protein: 3gm; Carbs: 5g; Fat: 7g

62. Rosemary Chicken

Preparation time: ten mins
Cooking time: ten mins
Servings: two
Ingredients:

- two zucchinis
- one carrot
- one tsp dried rosemary
- 4 chicken breasts
- half bell pepper
- half red onion
- 8 garlic cloves
- Olive oil
- quarter tbsp ground pepper

Directions:

1. Prepare the oven and preheat it at 375 °F (or 200°C).
2. Slice both zucchini and carrots and include bell pepper, onion, garlic, and put everything including oil in a 13" x 9" pan.
3. Spread the pepper over everything and roast for almost ten mins.
4. In the meantime, lift the chicken skin and spread black pepper and rosemary on the flesh.
5. Take away the vegetable pan from the oven and include the chicken, returning it to the oven for almost 30 more mins. Serve and relish!

Per serving: Calories: 215kcal; Protein: 2g; Carbs: 4g; Fat: 6.3g

63. Cinnamon Chicken Pesto Pasta

Preparation time: ten mins
Cooking time: ten mins, plus chilling time
Servings: 6
Ingredients:

- one teacup chicken breast, cubed cooked
- three teacups brown rice fusilli
- one teacup pistachio pesto
- one teacup plain low-fat milk
- one tsp cinnamon
- one tbsp crushed scallion
- one tbsp fresh orange juice
- half tsp salt
- quarter tsp freshly ground black pepper

Directions:

1. Cook the pasta following the package guidelines and drain and then place to a big container.
2. Whisk in the chicken, pistachio pesto, milk, cinnamon, scallion, orange juice, salt, and pepper. Toss till thoroughly blended.
3. Chilled prior to serving.

Per serving: Calories: 286kcal; Protein: 20g; Carbs: 26g; Fat: 12g

64. Roasted Chicken

Preparation time: sixty mins
Cooking time: sixty mins
Servings: eight
Ingredients:

- half tsp thyme
- three lbs. whole chicken
- one bay leaf
- three garlic pieces
- four tbsps coarsely severed orange peel
- half tsp black pepper
- half tbsp salt

Directions:

1. Bring the chicken to room temp. and let it sit for approximately one hr.
2. Utilizing the paper towels, thoroughly dry the interior as well as the exterior of the chicken.
3. Once you begin making the chicken seasoning, turn the oven temp. up to 450 degrees Fahrenheit.
4. Inside a separate container, mix the thyme, salt, and pepper together.
5. Use one-third of the seasoning for wiping the interior of the. Place the garlic, citrus peel, and bay leaf within the chicken before cooking.
6. Bind the legs together and tuck the tips of the wings into the body. After applying the remaining spice to the chicken, place it on a roasting pot. Roast the chicken.
7. Place in the oven and bake for one hour at a temp. of 160 degrees Fahrenheit.
8. Put away to rest for a quarter of an hour.
9. After the chicken has been roasted, cut it up and serve it.
10. Relish.

Per serving: Calories: 201kcal; Protein: 35.4g; Carbs: 0.8g; Fat: 5.3g

FISH-BASED RECIPES

65. SEARED GARLICKY COCONUT SCALLOPS 56
66. HONEY SCALLOPS 56
67. GARLIC COD MEAL 57
68. SAUTÉ LEMON-CAPER TROUT 57
69. FRESH MUSSELS IN COCONUT HERB BROTH 58
70. CABBAGE WITH ANCHOVIES 58
71. COCONUT CHILI SALMON 59
72. KALE COD SECRET 59
73. SALMON BROCCOLI BOWL 60
74. HERBED MUSSELS TREAT 60
75. FISH STICKS WITH AVOCADO DIPPING SAUCE 61
76. SOUP OF OYSTERS AND MUSHROOMS 62
77. AHI POKE WITH CUCUMBER 62
78. COCONUT-CRUSTED SHRIMP 63

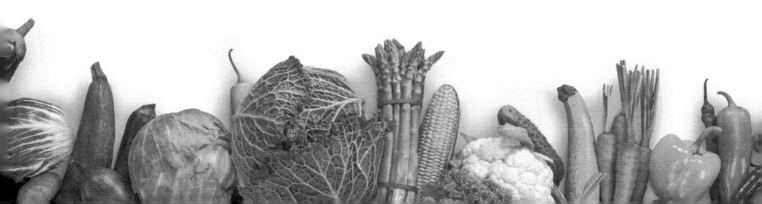

65. Seared Garlicky Coconut Scallops

Preparation time: ten mins
Cooking time: fifteen mins
Servings: 4
Ingredients:

- one lb. large scallops, washed
- Dash salt
- Dash freshly ground black pepper
- two tbsps avocado oil
- two garlic pieces, crushed
- three tbsps coconut aminos
- quarter teacup raw honey
- one tbsp apple cider vinegar

Directions:

1. Use paper towels to pat dry the scallops and spray with the salt and pepper.
2. Heat the avocado oil in a huge griddle at medium-high temp.
3. Include the scallops, then cook for two to three mins per side till golden. Transfer to a plate, use aluminum foil tent loosely to keep warm, and put away.
4. Include the garlic, coconut aminos, honey and vinegar into the same griddle, stir them together. Bring to a simmer, then cook for seven mins, blending irregularly as the liquid reduces.
5. Place the scallops back to the griddle with the glaze. Gently toss to coat and serve warm.

Per serving: Calories: 383kcal; Protein: 21g; Carbs: 26gm; Fat: 19g

66. Honey Scallops

Preparation time: five mins
Cooking time: twenty-five mins
Servings: four
Ingredients:

- one lb. large scallops, washed
- Dash of ground black pepper and salt as required
- three tbsps coconut aminos
- two garlic pieces, crushed
- two tbsps avocado oil
- quarter teacup raw honey
- one tbsp apple cider vinegar

Directions:

1. Spray the scallops with the salt and pepper.
2. In a griddle (you can also use a saucepan); warm the oil over medium stove flame.
3. Include the scallops, stir the solution and cook while mixing for almost two-three mins till softened and golden.
4. Transfer to a plate, and put away.
5. In the same griddle or pan, heat the honey, coconut aminos, garlic, and vinegar.
6. Cook for six-seven mins; include the scallops and coat well. Serve warm.

Per serving: Calories: 346kcal; Protein: 21g; Carbs: 27g; Fat: 17g

67. Garlic Cod Meal

Preparation time: five mins
Cooking time: thirty-five mins
Servings: four
Ingredients:

- two tbsps olive oil
- two tbsps tarragon, severed
- quarter teacup parsley, severed
- four cod fillets, skinless
- three garlic pieces, crushed
- one yellow onion, severed
- Ground black pepper and salt as required
- Juice of 1 lemon
- 1 lemon, (cut into slices)
- one tbsp thyme, severed
- four teacups water

Directions:

1. In a griddle (you can also use a saucepan); warm the oil over medium stove flame.
2. Include the onions, garlic, stir the solution and cook while mixing for almost two-three mins till softened.
3. Include the salt, pepper, tarragon, parsley, thyme, water, lemon juice and lemon slices.
4. Boil the mix; include the cod, cook for twelve-fifteen mins, drain the liquid.
5. Serve with a side salad.

Per serving: Calories: 181kcal; Protein: 12g; Carbs: 9g; Fat: 3g

68. Sauté Lemon-Caper Trout

Preparation time: ten mins
Cooking time: twenty mins
Servings: two
Ingredients:

For the Shallots

- one tsp coconut oil
- two shallots, finely cut
- Dash salt

For the Trout

- one tbsp plus one tsp coconut oil, split
- two (four-oz.) trout fillets
- quarter tsp salt
- quarter teacup freshly lemon juice, squeezed
- three tbsps capers
- Dash freshly ground black pepper
- one lemon, finely cut

Directions:

TO MAKE THE SHALLOTS

1. In a huge griddle, warm at middling temp. to cook the coconut oil, shallots, and salt about twenty mins, blending irregularly, till the shallots caramelized.

TO MAKE THE TROUT

2. When the shallots cook, in another griddle, warm at middling temp. to heat one tsp of coconut oil.
3. Place the trout fillets, cook for three mins per side, till the center is flaky, remove to a plate, put away.
4. Mix the salt, pepper, lemon juice, and capers together in the same griddle that you cooked the trout in. Stir in the rest of the one tbsp of coconut oil until the mixture is brought to a simmer. The fish should be served with the sauce.
5. If you choose, garnish the fish with the lemon slices and the shallots that have been caramelized.
6. Enjoy.

Per serving: Calories: 399kcal; Protein: 21g; Carbs: 17g; Fat: 22g

69. Fresh Mussels in Coconut Herb Broth

Preparation time: fifteen mins
Cooking time: fifteen mins
Servings: four
Ingredients:

- one tbsp olive oil
- 1½ pounds fresh mussels, scrubbed and debearded
- one teacup canned unsweetened coconut milk
- half teacup herbed chicken bone broth
- two tsps bottled crushed garlic
- two tsps severed fresh thyme
- one tsp severed fresh oregano
- 1 scallion, white & green parts, finely cut on an angle

Directions:

1. Heat the olive oil in your huge griddle at medium-high temp.
2. Place the garlic into the griddle. Sauté till softened, around three mins.
3. Include the chicken broth, coconut milk, oregano and thyme. Raise to a boil.
4. Stir in the mussels. Cover the griddle and steam till the shells open, about eight mins. Discard any unopened shells and remove the griddle from the heat.
5. Include the scallion and stir well. Serve instantly.

Per serving: Calories: 321kcal; Protein: 22g; Carbs: 11gm; Fat: 22g

70. Cabbage with Anchovies

Preparation time: ten mins
Cooking time: zero mins
Servings: two
Ingredients:

- two teacups of boiled cabbage
- two tbsps of capers
- 5 anchovies in oil
- 2 tomatoes
- 1 chili
- two tbsps of olive oil
- one tweak of salt
- one tweak of cayenne pepper
- one tbsp of severed fresh parsley

Directions:

1. Inside a container, mix thoroughly the anchovies cut into small pieces, the severed chili pepper, the parsley, the whole capers, the cubed tomatoes, the oil, the salt, the pepper.
2. Include the cabbage and mix again.

Per serving: Calories: 257kcal; Protein: 12g; Carbs: 11g; Fat: 19g

71. Coconut Chili Salmon

Preparation time: ten mins
Cooking time: twenty-five mins
Servings: 6
Ingredients:

- one and quarter teacups coconut, shredded
- two tbsps olive oil
- quarter teacup water
- one lb. salmon, cubed
- one-third teacup coconut flour
- a tweak of (ground) black pepper and salt
- one egg
- 4 red chilies, severed
- three garlic pieces, crushed
- quarter teacup balsamic vinegar
- half teacup raw honey

Directions:

1. Inside a container (medium size), mix the flour with a tweak of salt.
2. Inside a separate container, whisk the egg and black pepper.
3. Include the shredded coconut in another container.
4. Coat the salmon cubes in flour, egg and coconut mix one by one.
5. In a griddle (you can also use a saucepan); warm the oil over medium stove flame.
6. Include the salmon, stir-fry them for 2-three mins on all sides. Place in serving plates.
7. Heat water at medium-high temp. in the pan, include the chilies, cloves, vinegar and honey, stir gently.
8. Boil the mix and simmer for four mins; top over the salmon and serve.

Per serving: Calories: 218kcal; Protein: 17g; Carbs: 14g; Fat: 5g

72. Kale Cod Secret

Preparation time: ten mins
Cooking time: thirty mins
Servings: four
Ingredients:

- four cod fillets, skinless and boneless
- one tbsp ginger, (shredded or grated)
- 4 teaspoons lemon zest
- a tweak of (ground) black pepper and salt
- 3 leeks, severed
- two teacups veggie stock
- two tbsps lemon juice
- two tbsps olive oil
- one lb. kale, severed
- half tsp sesame oil

Directions:

1. Inside a container (medium size), mix the zest with salt and pepper. Coat the fish with this mix.
2. In a griddle (you can also use a saucepan); heat the leeks, ginger and lemon juice over medium stove flame.
3. Heat for a few minutes; include the fish fillets.
4. Cover and cook for eight-ten mins, transfer it to a plate.
5. Strain the liquid and reserve the leeks. Include the fish in serving plates.
6. In a griddle (you can also use a saucepan); warm the oil over medium stove flame.
7. Include the kale, stir the solution and cook while mixing for almost three-four mins till softened.
8. Include the soup liquid and cook for 4-five mins more.
9. Include the reserved leeks; cook for two mins.
10. Split into fish containers, drizzle the sesame oil all over and serve.

Per serving: Calories: 238kcal; Protein: 16g; Carbs: 12gm; Fat: 3gm

73. Salmon Broccoli Bowl

Preparation time: five mins
Cooking time: twenty mins
Servings: four
Ingredients:

- three tbsps avocado oil
- two garlic pieces, crushed
- 1 broccoli head, separate florets
- one and half lbs.s salmon fillets, boneless
- A tweak of (ground) black pepper and salt
- Juice of ½ lemon

Directions:

1. Warm up an oven to 450°F. Line a baking sheet with a foil.
2. Spread the broccoli; include the salmon, oil, garlic, salt, pepper and the lemon juice, toss gently.
3. Bake for fifteen mins.
4. Split in serving plates and serve warm.

Per serving: Calories: 207kcal; Protein: 9g; Carbs: 14g; Fat: 6g

74. Herbed Mussels Treat

Preparation time: five mins
Cooking time: thirty mins
Servings: four
Ingredients:

- one tbsp olive oil
- two tsps crushed garlic
- one teacup coconut milk
- half teacup chicken bone broth
- two tsps severed fresh thyme
- one tsp severed fresh oregano
- one and half lbs. mussels, scrubbed and debearded
- 1 scallion, sliced white and green parts

Directions:

1. In a griddle (you can also use a saucepan); warm the oil over medium stove flame.
2. Include the garlic, stir the solution and cook while mixing for almost two-three mins till softened.
3. Include the coconut milk, broth, thyme, and oregano.
4. Boil the mix and include the mussels. Cover and cook for almost eight mins, or till the shells opened up.
5. Take out any unopened shells and include in the scallion; serve warm.

Per serving: Calories: 318kcal; Protein: 23g; Carbs: 12g; Fat: 21g

75. Fish Sticks with Avocado Dipping Sauce

Preparation time: fifteen mins
Cooking time: five mins
Servings: four
Ingredients:

For the avocado dipping sauce

- 2 avocados
- quarter teacup lime juice
- two tbsps fresh cilantro leaves
- two tbsps olive oil
- one tsp salt
- one tsp garlic powder
- Dash ground cumin
- Black pepper

For the fish sticks

- one and half teacups almond flour
- one tsp salt
- half tsp paprika
- quarter tsp black pepper
- 3 eggs
- quarter teacup coconut oil
- one lb. cod fillets, cut into 4-inch-long, 1-inch-thick strips
- Juice of one lemon

Directions:

1. In a suitable blending container, blend the avocados, lime juice, cilantro, olive oil, salt, garlic powder, and cumin, and flavour with pepper till smooth
2. In a small shallow container, mix the almond flour, salt, paprika, and pepper. Whisk the eggs in another small shallow container.
3. Dip the fish sticks into the egg and then into the almond flour solution till fully coated.
4. In a suitable griddle at medium-high temp., heat the coconut oil.
5. One at a time, place the fish sticks in the griddle. Cook for almost two mins on all sides till lightly browned. Apportion them between 2 plates.
6. To serve, spray with the lemon juice and serve alongside the avocado dipping sauce.

Per serving: Calories: 583kcal; Protein: 25g; Carbs: 14g; Fat: 50g

76. Soup of Oysters and Mushrooms

Preparation time: ten mins
Cooking time: fifty mins
Servings: six
Ingredients:

- 15 oysters
- one tsp of oregano
- one tsp of thyme
- one teacup of white mushrooms
- two teacups low sodium vegetable broth
- one onion
- one leek
- one yellow potato
- one tbsp of coconut butter

Directions:

1. In a non-stick pan, dissolve the coconut butter and brown the severed onion and leek.
2. Include the sliced mushrooms, mix and after a minute include the vegetable broth and cook for twenty mins over moderate heat.
3. Include the thyme and oregano.
4. Cut the potato into cubes, include it and cook for another twenty mins.
5. Wash the oysters well, put them in a saucepan with the lid on low heat to make them open.
6. Once opened, extract the mollusks and filter the liquid they have released with a strainer.
7. Include the liquid to the mushrooms and potatoes.
8. Cook for another three mins, include the oysters, mix and serve.

Per serving: Calories: 101kcal; Protein: 7g; Carbs: 9g; Fat: 8g

77. Ahi Poke with Cucumber

Preparation time: twenty mins
Cooking time: zero mins
Servings: four
Ingredients:

- one lb. (454 g) sushi-grade ahi tuna, cut into one-inch cubes
- three scallions, finely cut
- one serrano chili, sowed and crushed (optional)
- three tbsps coconut aminos
- one tsp rice vinegar
- one tsp sesame oil
- one tsp toasted sesame seeds
- Dash ground ginger
- one big avocado, cubed
- one cucumber, sliced into half inch-thick rounds

Directions:

1. In a big container, gently mix the first eight components till thoroughly blended.
2. Cover and refrigerate to marinate for fifteen mins.
3. Stir in the avocado, gently incorporating the chunks into the ahi solution.
4. Organize the cucumber slices on a plate.
5. Put a spoonful of the ahi poke on every cucumber slice and serve instantly.

Per serving: Calories: 214kcal; Protein: 10g; Carbs: 11g; Fat: 15g

78. Coconut-Crusted Shrimp

Preparation time: ten mins
Cooking time: six mins
Servings: four
Ingredients:

- 2 eggs
- one teacup unsweetened dried coconut
- quarter teacup coconut flour
- half tsp salt
- quarter tsp paprika
- Dash cayenne pepper
- Dash black pepper
- quarter teacup coconut oil
- one lb. raw shrimp, skinned and deveined

Directions:

1. In a small shallow container, beat all the eggs.
2. In another small shallow container, mix the coconut, coconut flour, salt, paprika, cayenne pepper, and black pepper.
3. In a suitable griddle, heat the coconut oil at medium-high temp..
4. Pat the shrimp dry with a paper towel.
5. Working one at a time, hold each shrimp by the tail, dip it into the egg solution, and then into the coconut solution till coated. Place into the hot griddle. Cook for almost three mins on all sides.
6. Transfer the hot shrimp to a paper towel-lined plate to drain extra oil.
7. Serve instantly.

Per serving: Calories: 279kcal; Protein: 19g; Carbs: 6g; Fat: 20g

VEGETARIAN RECIPES

- 79. Ginger Carrot and Pineapple Juice 65
- 80. Buckwheat Lemon Tabbouleh 65
- 81. Sauté Lentil Sloppy Joes 66
- 82. Pesto Portobello Mushroom Burger 66
- 83. Fresh Spring Roll Wraps 67
- 84. Stir-Fried Squash 67
- 85. Mushroom Tacos 68
- 86. Curried Okra 68
- 87. Turmeric Endives 69
- 88. Cauliflower Hash Brown 69
- 89. Roasted Seasoned Carrots 70
- 90. Braised Kale 70
- 91. Sweet Potato Puree 71

79. Ginger Carrot and Pineapple Juice

Preparation time: ten mins
Cooking time: zero mins
Servings: two
Ingredients:

- 8 carrots, roughly severed
- one (one inch) piece skinned fresh ginger
- three teacups severed fresh pineapple
- quarter teacup filtered water
- Ice, for serving

Directions:

1. Include the carrots, ginger, pineapple and water into a mixer, blend till smooth.
2. Set over the top of a medium container with a nut milk bag or piece of cheesecloth. Pour the juice into the mesh material. Squeeze to drain well. Discard the solids.
3. Pour the juice in two tall glasses, include ice and serve instantly.

Per serving: Calories: 135kcal; Protein: 2.6g; Carbs: 40g; Fat: 0.7g

80. Buckwheat Lemon Tabbouleh

Preparation time: fifteen mins
Cooking time: ten mins
Servings: four
Ingredients:

- one tbsp olive oil
- two tsps bottled crushed garlic
- half teacup severed red onion
- Juice of one lemon (three tbsps)
- two teacups cooked buckwheat
- Zest of one lemon (optional)
- quarter teacup severed fresh mint
- half teacup severed fresh parsley
- Sea salt

Directions:

1. Place a large griddle at medium-high temp. and begin to warm the olive oil in the pan.
2. Include the garlic and the red onion and stir to combine. Sauté till transparent, around three mins.
3. Include the juice of one lemon, the buckwheat, and the zest of one lemon (if utilizing). For around five mins, sauté the meat till it is completely heated through.
4. After adding the mint and parsley, give the mixture a good toss and continue to sauté for extra min.
5. Take off the heat and season with a pinch of salt from the sea.

Per serving: Calories: 184kcal; Protein: 6g; Carbs: 34g; Fat: 5g

81. Sauté Lentil Sloppy Joes

Preparation time: ten mins
Cooking time: twenty mins
Servings: four
Ingredients:

- two tbsps avocado oil, split
- one small white onion, severed
- one celery stalk, finely severed
- one carrot, crushed
- two garlic pieces, crushed
- one lb. cooked lentils
- ½ red bell pepper, finely severed
- 7 tbsps. tomato paste
- two tbsps apple cider vinegar
- one tbsp pure maple syrup
- one tsp Dijon mustard
- one tsp chili powder
- half tsp dried oregano

Directions:

1. Inside a pot, warm at medium-high temp. to heat one tbsp of avocado oil.
2. Blend the onion, celery, carrot, and garlic, sauté for almost three mins, 'til the onion is translucent.
3. Place the lentils and the remaining one tbsp of avocado oil, sauté for almost five mins.
4. Place the red bell pepper, sauté for two mins.
5. Mix in the tomato paste, vinegar, maple syrup, mustard, chili powder, and oregano. Decrease the temp. to medium-low then cook for almost ten mins, blending irregularly.
6. Serve on gluten-free bread or over rice.

Per serving: Calories: 277kcal; Protein: 14g; Carbs: 29g; Fat: 7g

82. Pesto Portobello Mushroom Burger

Preparation time: five mins
Cooking time: twenty mins
Servings: four
Ingredients:

- four tomato slices
- four onion slices
- 4 portobello mushroom caps, stemmed, gills removed
- 1 spinach pesto
- 4 whole-wheat hamburger buns

Directions:

1. Warm up the oven to 400 deg. F.
2. Use pesto to brush the both sides of mushroom caps to coat and transfer them onto a rimmed baking sheet. Bake till soft, about fifteen to twenty mins.
3. On the buns layer with the mushrooms along with the onions and tomatoes. Serve.

Per serving: Calories: 339kcal; Protein: 12g; Carbs: 26g; Fat: 23g

83. Fresh Spring Roll Wraps

Preparation time: twenty mins
Cooking time: one min
Servings: four to six
Ingredients:

- two teacups lightly packed baby spinach, split
- one teacup grated carrot, split
- one cucumber, shared, sowed, and cut into thin, 4-inch-long strips, split
- 1 avocado, shared, pitted, and cut into thin strips, split
- 10 rice paper wrappers

Directions:

1. Find a flat surface to place a cutting board, put the vegetables in front of you.
2. Fill warm water into a large, shallow container—hot enough to cook the wrappers, but warm enough so you can touch it comfortably. Soak 1 wrapper in the water and then place it on the cutting board.
3. Fill quarter teacup of spinach, two tbsps of grated carrot, a few cucumber slices, and 1 or 2 slices of avocado in the middle of the wrapper.
4. Fold the sides over the middle, and then tightly roll the wrapper from the bottom, burrito-style.
5. Repeat with the remaining wrappers and vegetables.
6. After done, serve instantly.

Per serving: Calories: 246kcal; Protein: 4g; Carbs: 36gm; Fat: 10g

84. Stir-Fried Squash

Preparation time: ten mins
Cooking time: ten mins
Servings: four
Ingredients:

- one tbsp olive oil
- three pieces of garlic, crushed
- one butternut squash, sowed and sliced
- one tbsp coconut aminos
- one tbsp lemon juice
- one tbsp water
- Salt and pepper as required

Directions:

1. Bring the oil at a medium temp., add the garlic, and cook it till it becomes fragrant.
2. After the squash has been stirred in for the previous three mins, proceed to include the remaining components.
3. Replace the cover and continue to cook the squash for a further five mins, or till it reaches the desired consistency.
4. Serve, and have fun with it!

Per serving: Calories: 83kcal; Protein: 2g; Carbs: 14g; Fat: 3g

85. Mushroom Tacos

Preparation time: ten mins
Cooking time: fifteen mins
Servings: six
Ingredients:

- six collard greens leave
- two teacups mushrooms, severed
- 2 white onion, cubed
- two tbsps taco flavouring
- two tbsps coconut oil
- half tsp salt
- quarter teacup fresh parsley
- two tbsps mayonnaise

Directions:

1. Put the coconut oil in the griddle and dissolve it.
2. Include severed mushrooms and cubed onion. Mix up the components.
3. Close the lid and cook them for ten mins.
4. After this, spray the vegetables with Taco flavouring, salt, and include fresh parsley.
5. Mix up the solution and cook for five mins more.
6. Then include mayonnaise and stir well.
7. Chill the mushroom solution a little.
8. Fill the collard green leaves with the mushroom solution and fold up them.

Per serving: Calories: 52kcal; Protein: 1.4g; Carbs: 5.1g; Fat: 3.3g

86. Curried Okra

Preparation time: ten mins
Cooking time: twelve mins
Servings: four
Ingredients:

- one lb. small to medium okra pods, clipped
- quarter tsp curry powder
- half tsp kosher salt
- one tsp finely severed serrano chili
- one tsp ground coriander
- one tbsp canola oil
- three-quarter tsp brown mustard seeds

Directions:

1. Put a big and heavy griddle over a temp. that is medium-high, and sauté the mustard seeds till aromatic, which should take almost thirty secs.
2. Include canola oil. Include okra in the dish along with curry powder, salt, chile, and ground coriander. Stir the mixture occasionally whilst cooking it for one min on a sauté pan.
3. Place a cover on the pan and continue to simmer at a low flame for almost eight mins. Mix it up every so often.
4. Take out the cover, raise the heat to medium-high, and continue cooking the okra for around extra two mins, or till it has a light brown color.
5. Serve and relish.

Per serving: Calories: 78kcal; Protein: 2g; Carbs: 6g; Fat: 6g

87. Turmeric Endives

Preparation time: ten mins
Cooking time: twenty mins
Servings: four
Ingredients:

- two endives, shared lengthwise
- two tbsps olive oil
- one tsp rosemary, dried
- half tsp turmeric powder
- A tweak of black pepper

Directions:

1. Mix the endives with the oil and the other components in a baking pan, toss gently, bake at 400 degrees F within twenty mins.
2. Serve as a side dish.

Per serving: Calories: 64kcal; Protein: 0.2g; Carbs: 0.8g; Fat: 7.1g

88. Cauliflower Hash Brown

Preparation time: ten mins
Cooking time: twenty mins
Servings: six
Ingredients:

- four eggs, whisked
- half teacup coconut milk
- half tsp dry mustard
- Salt and pepper as required
- one big head cauliflower, shredded

Directions:

1. Blend the entire components inside a blending dish and stir till everything is evenly distributed.
2. Warm up a frypan that does not require oil or butter at a moderate temp.
3. Place a sizeable scoop of the cauliflower solution in the center of the hot griddle.
4. Fry one side for three mins, then turn it and fry the other side for one min, just like you would with a pancake. Proceed with the other components in the same manner.
5. Serve and relish.

Per serving: Calories: 102kcal; Protein: 5g; Carbs: 4g; Fat: 8g

89. Roasted Seasoned Carrots

Preparation time: fifteen mins
Cooking time: twenty mins
Servings: four
Ingredients:

- 8 carrots, skinned and cut into half inch-wide and 3-inch-long sticks
- two tbsps olive oil, plus more for greasing the baking sheet
- quarter tsp dried dill
- one tsp dried parsley
- quarter tsp onion powder
- one tsp garlic powder
- Tweak of sea salt
- one tbsp severed fresh dill

Directions:

1. Warm up the oven to 400 deg. F.
2. Use olive oil to lightly grease a rimmed baking sheet, set it aside.
3. Include the dill, parsley, onion powder, garlic powder and sea salt into a small container, stir them together.
4. On the baking sheet, spread the carrots. Sprinkle the flavouring mix over and drizzle with the remaining two tbsps of olive oil.
5. Roast the carrots till lightly caramelized and soft, about twenty mins. Place to a serving container, garnish with the fresh dill, and serve.

Per serving: Calories: 115kcal; Protein: 1g; Carbs: 13gm; Fat: 7g

90. Braised Kale

Preparation time: ten mins
Cooking time: fifteen mins
Servings: three
Ingredients:

- two-three tbsps water
- one tbsp coconut oil
- half sliced red pepper
- two stalk celery (sliced to quarter inch thick)
- five teacups of severed kale

Directions:

1. Bring a skillet to a temp. of middling temp.
2. After the celery has been sautéed in the olive oil for almost five mins, include the coconut oil.
3. Put the greens and the red pepper in the pan.
4. Pour one tbsp of water into the mixture.
5. Give the vegetables a couple of mins for wilting in the heat. If the kale begins to stick to the pot, include one tbsp of water to the mixture.
6. Serve while still hot.

Per serving: Calories: 61kcal; Protein: 1g; Carbs: 3g; Fat: 5g

91. Sweet Potato Puree

Preparation time: ten mins
Cooking time: fifteen mins
Servings: five
Ingredients:

- two lbs. sweet potatoes, skinned
- one and half teacups water
- five medjool dates, pitted and severed

Directions:

1. Start by placing potatoes and water in a pot.
2. Replace the top and continue to boil the potatoes for a minimum of fifteen mins, or till they are tender.
3. After draining the potatoes, throw them in the container of a blending container collectively with the dates.
4. Beat till the mixture is even.
5. Serve and relish.

Per serving: Calories: 172kcal; Protein: 3g; Carbs: 41g; Fat: 0.2g

VEGAN RECIPES

92. Cauliflower Mashed Potatoes 73
93. Paprika Brussels Sprouts 73
94. Baked Sweet Potatoes with Tomatoes 74
95. Zucchini Arugula and Olive Salad 75
96. Easy Slow Cooker Caramelized Onions 75
97. Spicy Wasabi Mayonnaise 76
98. Stir-Fried Almond and Spinach 76
99. Roasted Portobellos with Rosemary 76
100. Vegetable Potpie 77
101. Cilantro and Avocado Platter 77
102. Onion and Orange Healthy Salad 78
103. Broccoli with Garlic and Lemon 78

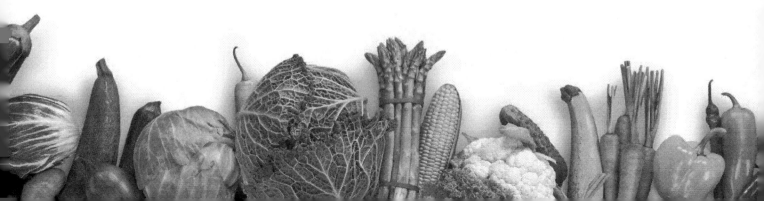

92. Cauliflower Mashed Potatoes

Preparation time: ten mins
Cooking time: ten mins
Servings: four
Ingredients:

- sixteen teacups water (sufficient to cover cauliflower)
- one head cauliflower (around three lbs), clipped and cut into florets
- four garlic pieces
- one tbsp olive oil
- quarter tsp salt
- one-eighth tsp freshly ground black pepper
- two tsps dried parsley

Directions:

1. Bring a big saucepan of water to a boil, then add the garlic and cauliflower to the pot. After ten mins of cooking, drain the liquid. After moving it back to the heated pot, cover it and allow it stand for two to three mins prior to serving.
2. Place the cauliflower and garlic in a blending container or mixer and process until smooth. Include the olive oil, salt, and pepper, and then purée the mixture until it is smooth. Examine the seasonings and make any necessary adjustments.
3. Take out, then replace with the parsley, and continue mixing until everything is incorporated. If you like, you can finish the dish off with a drizzle of additional olive oil. Instantly serve after cooking.

Per serving: Calories: 87kcal; Protein: 4g; Carbs: 12g; Fat: 4g

93. Paprika Brussels Sprouts

Preparation time: ten mins
Cooking time: twenty-five mins
Servings: four
Ingredients:

- two tbsps olive oil
- one lb. brussels sprouts, clipped and shared
- three green onions, severed
- two garlic pieces, crushed
- one tbsp balsamic vinegar
- one tbsp sweet paprika
- A tweak of black pepper

Directions:

1. Inside a baking pot, blend the Brussels sprouts with the oil and the remaining components, toss and bake at 400 deg. F within twenty-five mins.
2. Split the mix between plates and serve.

Per serving: Calories: 121kcal; Protein: 4.4g; Carbs: 12.6g; Fat: 7.6g

94. Baked Sweet Potatoes with Tomatoes

Preparation time: five mins whilst the sweet potatoes bake
Cooking time: twenty-five mins
Servings: four
Ingredients:

- four medium sweet potatoes
- one tbsp avocado oil
- two garlic pieces, crushed
- one small white onion, finely cut
- one (fourteen oz.) can black beans, drained & washed well
- quarter tsp red pepper flakes
- twelve cherry tomatoes, severed
- half tsp chili powder
- quarter tsp salt
- one big avocado, sliced
- Juice of one lime

Directions:

1. Set the oven temp. to 400 degrees Fahrenheit.
2. Using a fork, pierce every sweet potato a total of five times to create holes. Bake the sweet potatoes for twenty-five mins after wrapping each one in a piece of aluminum foil and placing them on a baking pan.
3. Whilst that is happening, warm the avocado oil in a sauté pot at a moderate flame. Mix the garlic and onion together, then cook them for five mins.
4. After mixing in the beans, red pepper flakes, tomatoes, chili powder, and salt, continue to simmer the mixture for approximately seven mins. Retrieve from the burning.
5. When the sweet potatoes are done cooking, take them out from the oven and get rid of the aluminum foil from around them. Cut every potato in half lengthwise, then slice them almost all the way across to the bottom.
6. Cut the potatoes in half lengthwise to make room for the filling, and then place a comparable quantity of the filling in each potato half.
7. Garnish with slices of avocado and a little spray of lime juice.

Per serving: Calories: 326kcal; Protein: 10g; Carbs: 51g; Fat: 10g

95. Zucchini Arugula and Olive Salad

Preparation time: fifteen mins
Cooking time: zero mins
Servings: four
Ingredients:

- ½ small red onion, finely cut
- two large zucchinis, thinly sliced
- one teacup arugula
- half teacup pitted green olives, sliced
- 2 radishes, thinly sliced
- two tbsps fresh lemon juice
- two tbsps extra-virgin olive oil
- one-eighth tsp. red pepper flakes
- one tsp salt

Directions:

1. Include the red onion, zucchini, arugula, green olives and radishes into a medium container, blend them together.
2. Then mix in the lemon juice, olive oil, red pepper flakes and salt, toss to thoroughly blended.
3. Serve immediately.

Per serving: Calories: 120kcal; Protein: 2g; Carbs: 7g; Fat: 10g

96. Easy Slow Cooker Caramelized Onions

Preparation time: fifteen mins or fewer
Cooking time: 10 hrs on low
Servings: two teacups
Ingredients:

- two tbsps extra-virgin olive oil
- four large onions (white or sweet), sliced very thin
- half tsp sea salt

Directions:

1. Include the olive oil, onions and sea salt into the slow cooker, stir to cover the onions with the oil.
2. Cover the cooker and cook for 10 hours on low. Drain the liquid and serve.

Per serving: Calories: 234kcal; Protein: 3g; Carbs: 26gm; Fat: 14g

97. Spicy Wasabi Mayonnaise

Preparation time: fifteen mins
Cooking time: zero mins
Servings: four
Ingredients:

- half tbsp wasabi paste
- one teacup mayonnaise

Directions:

1. Grab a container and combine the mayonnaise and wasabi paste in it.
2. Give it a thorough combination.
3. Allow it to chill, then utilize it as required.
4. Serve, and have fun with it!

Per serving: Calories: 388kcal; Protein: 1g; Carbs: 1g; Fat: 42g

98. Stir-Fried Almond and Spinach

Preparation time: ten mins
Cooking time: fifteen mins
Servings: two
Ingredients:

- three-quarter lbs. spinach
- three tbsps almonds
- Salt as required
- one tbsp coconut oil

Directions:

1. In a big pot, add the oil, and then put the pot over a high temp.
2. After adding the spinach, continue to let it cook while mixing it constantly.
3. When the spinach is done cooking and has reached the desired tenderness, season it with salt and mix it.
4. Include almonds and relish!

Per serving: Calories: 150kcal; Protein: 8g; Carbs: 10g; Fat: 12g

99. Roasted Portobellos with Rosemary

Preparation time: five mins
Cooking time: fifteen mins
Servings: four
Ingredients:

- eight portobello mushroom, clipped
- one sprig rosemary, torn
- two tbsps fresh lemon juice
- quarter teacup extra virgin olive oil
- one piece garlic, crushed
- Salt and pepper, as required

Directions:

1. Set your oven to a temp. of 450° Fahrenheit and warm it.
2. Get a container and put the entire components in it.
3. Shake to cover everything.
4. Organize the mushrooms in a single layer on a baking tray with the stems facing up.
5. Place in the oven and roast for a total of fifteen mins.
6. Serve, and have fun with it!

Per serving: Calories: 63kcal; Protein: 1g; Carbs: 2g; Fat: 6g

100. Vegetable Potpie

Preparation time: ten mins
Cooking time: ten mins
Servings: eight
Ingredients:

- one recipe pastry for double-crust pie
- two tbsps cornstarch
- one tsp ground black pepper
- one tsp kosher salt
- three teacups vegetable broth
- one teacup fresh green beans, snapped into half inch
- two teacups cauliflower florets
- two stalks celery, sliced ¼ inch wide
- two potatoes, skinned and cubed
- two big carrots, cubed
- one piece garlic, crushed
- eight oz. mushroom
- one onion, severed
- two tbsps olive oil

Directions:

1. Inside a big saucepot, sauté the garlic in the oil till it is just beginning to brown. Include the onions and continue to sauté till the onions are luminous and tender.
2. Sauté the celery, potatoes, and carrots for three mins after adding them.
3. Put the cauliflower and green beans into the pot, along with the vegetable stock, and heat to a boil. Slow fire and simmer till vegetables are somewhat soft. Include some black pepper and salt as required.
4. Inside a small container, combine a quarter teacup of water with cornstarch. Continue to stir the solution till it is completely lump-free and even. After that, pour the mixture into the pot containing the vegetables whilst continuously mixing.
5. Keep mixing till the soup begins to dense, which should take almost three mins. Take away from the fire.
6. In the meantime, stretch out the pastry dough and set it on a baking tray that is safe for the oven measuring eleven by seven. After that, cover it with another layer of pastry dough and pour the veggie filling on top. Seal and flute the outermost portion of the dough, then use a fork to make multiple pricks in the top dough and move on to the next step.
7. Bake the dish in an oven that has been prepared to 425 degrees Fahrenheit for approximately thirty mins, or till the crust begins to take on a golden brown color.

Per serving: Calories: 202kcal; Protein: 4g; Carbs: 26g; Fat: 10g

101. Cilantro and Avocado Platter

Preparation time: ten mins
Cooking time: zero mins
Servings: six
Ingredients:

- two avocados, skinned, pitted and cubed
- one sweet onion, severed
- one green bell pepper, severed
- one big ripe tomato, severed
- quarter teacup of fresh cilantro, severed
- half a lime, juiced
- Salt and pepper as required

Directions:

1. Put the onion, bell pepper, tomato, avocados, lime, and cilantro within a container of a moderate size.
2. Giving it a good stir, then throw it about.
3. To suit your palate, flavour the dish with salt and pepper according to your preference.
4. Prepare, and savor every bite!

Per serving: Calories: 126kcal; Protein: 2g; Carbs: 10g; Fat: 10g

102. Onion and Orange Healthy Salad

Preparation time: ten mins
Cooking time: zero mins
Servings: three
Ingredients:

- six big orange
- three tbsps of red wine vinegar
- six tbsps of olive oil
- one tsp of dried oregano
- one red onion, thinly sliced
- one teacup olive oil
- quarter teacup of fresh chives, severed
- Ground black pepper

Directions:

1. Take out the skin from the oranges and cut each one into four to five slices going across.
2. Place the oranges in a dish that is not very deep.
3. Spray vinegar, olive oil and also spray oregano.
4. Throw.
5. Chill for a total of half an hour.
6. Distribute sliced onion and black olives across the top of the dish.
7. Garnish with a further dash of chopped chives and a generous amount of freshly ground black pepper.
8. Serve, and have fun with it!

Per serving: Calories: 120kcal; Protein: 2g; Carbs: 20g; Fat: 6g

103. Broccoli with Garlic and Lemon

Preparation time: two mins
Cooking time: four mins
Servings: four
Ingredients:

- one teacup of water
- four teacups broccoli florets
- one tsp olive oil
- one tbsp crushed garlic
- one tsp lemon zest
- Salt
- Freshly ground black pepper

Directions:

1. Put the broccoli in the boiling water in a small saucepan and cook within 2 to three mins. The broccoli should retain its bright-green color. Drain the water from the broccoli.
2. Put the olive oil in a small sauté pan at medium-high temp.. Include the garlic then sauté for thirty secs. Put the broccoli, lemon zest, salt, plus pepper. Blend well and serve.

Per serving: Calories: 38kcal; Protein: 3g; Carbs: 5g; Fat: 1g

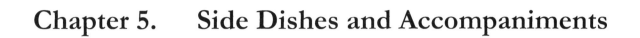

Chapter 5. Side Dishes and Accompaniments

Recipes

104. Salt & Vinegar Kale Crisps	80
105. Chili Broccoli	80
106. Lime Carrots	80
107. Tomato Bulgur	81
108. Green Beans	81
109. Basil Olives Mix	82
110. Lemon Asparagus	82
111. Mascarpone Couscous	82
112. Balsamic Cabbage	83
113. Spiced Nuts	83
114. Parmesan Endives	83
115. Fresh Strawberry Salsa	84
116. Roasted Carrots	84
117. Beet Hummus	84
118. Celery and Fennel Salad with Cranberries	85
119. Roasted Garlic Chickpeas	85
120. Roasted Parsnips	85
121. Crispy Corn	86
122. Easy Guacamole	86
123. Lima Beans Dish	87
124. Cashew "Humus"	87
125. Apple Crisp	88

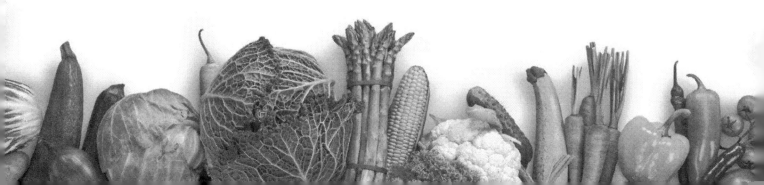

104. Salt & Vinegar Kale Crisps

Preparation time: five mins
Cooking time: twenty to twenty-five mins
Servings: two
Ingredients:

- four teacups kale, torn into two-inch parts
- two tbsps olive oil
- two tbsps apple cider vinegar
- one tsp sea salt, fine

Directions:

1. Put your oven on the middle rack and preheat it to 350 degrees. Bring out a container to use for mixing, and set the entire components in there.
2. Organize the kale in a single layer on a baking tray and bake it for twenty-five to thirty mins. Throw something at the midway point of this round.
3. Place in a container that can seal air out at room temp. They can be stored for up to two days.

Per serving: Calories: 135kcal; Protein: 1g; Carbs: 12g; Fat: 1g

105. Chili Broccoli

Preparation time: ten mins
Cooking time: thirty mins
Servings: four
Ingredients:

- two tbsps olive oil
- one lb. broccoli florets
- two garlic pieces, crushed
- two tbsps chili sauce
- one tbsp lemon juice
- A tweak of black pepper
- two tbsps cilantro, severed

Directions:

1. Inside a baking pot, blend the broccoli with the oil, garlic, and the other, toss a bit, and bake at 400 degrees F for thirty mins.
2. Split the mix between plates and serve as a side dish.

Per serving: Calories: 103kcal; Protein: 3.4g; Carbs: 8.3g; Fat: 7.4g

106. Lime Carrots

Preparation time: ten mins
Cooking time: thirty mins
Servings: four
Ingredients:

- one lb. baby carrots, clipped
- one tbsp sweet paprika
- one tsp lime juice
- three tbsps olive oil
- a tweak of black pepper
- one tsp sesame seeds

Directions:

1. Organize the carrots on a lined baking sheet, include the paprika and the other components excluding the sesame seeds, toss, bake at 400 degrees F within thirty mins.
2. Split the carrots among plates, spray sesame seeds on top and serve as a side dish.

Per serving: Calories: 139kcal; Protein: 1.1g; Carbs: 10.5g; Fat: 11.2g

107. Tomato Bulgur

Preparation time: seven mins
Cooking time: twenty mins
Servings: two
Ingredients:

- half teacup bulgur
- one tsp tomato paste
- half white onion, cubed
- two tbsps coconut oil
- one and half teacups chicken stock

Directions:

1. Place the coconut oil into a saucepan and stir until it is melted.
2. Include onion cubes and roast them until they are a light brown color.
3. After that, add the bulgur and give it a good toss.
4. Prepare the bulgur by cooking it for three mins in coconut oil.
5. After that, incorporate the tomato paste and thoroughly combine the bulgur until it is uniform.
6. Be sure to add chicken stock.
7. Put the top back on the pot and let the bulgur cook for fifteen mins at a temp. that is about average.
8. The finished bulgur ought to be allowed to absorb most of the liquid.

Per serving: Calories: 257kcal; Protein: 5.2g; Carbs: 30.2g; Fat: 14.5g

108. Green Beans

Preparation time: five mins
Cooking time: ten mins
Servings: five
Ingredients:

- half tsp of red pepper flakes
- two tbsps of extra-virgin olive oil
- two garlic pieces, crushed
- one and half lbs. green beans, clipped
- two tbsps of water
- half tsp kosher salt

Directions:

1. Bring the oil to a temp. of about moderate in a frying pan.
2. Don't forget to add the pepper flakes. Olive oil should be stirred in to ensure a coating.
3. Don't forget to add the green beans. Wait seven mins prior to serving.
4. Stir regularly. There ought to be some browning on the bean surfaces.
5. Season with salt and mince the garlic. Stirring constantly, cook the mixture for one min.
6. After pouring the water, instantly put the lid back on.
7. Continue cooking with the lid on for additional one min.

Per serving: Calories: 82kcal; Protein: 1g; Carbs: 6g; Fat: 6g

109. Basil Olives Mix

Preparation time: five mins
Cooking time: zero mins
Servings: four
Ingredients:

- two tbsps olive oil
- one tbsp balsamic vinegar
- A tweak of black pepper
- four teacups corn
- two teacups black olives, pitted and shared
- one red onion, severed
- half teacup cherry tomatoes shared
- one tbsp basil, severed
- one tbsp jalapeno, severed
- two teacups romaine lettuce, shredded

Directions:

1. Mix the corn with the olives, lettuce, and the other components in a big container, toss thoroughly, split between plates and serve as a side dish.

Per serving: Calories: 290kcal; Protein: 6.2g; Carbs: 37.6gm; Fat: 16.1g

110. Lemon Asparagus

Preparation time: ten mins
Cooking time: twenty mins
Servings: four
Ingredients:

- one lb. asparagus, clipped
- two tbsps basil pesto
- one tbsp lemon juice
- A tweak of black pepper
- three tbsps olive oil
- two tbsps cilantro, severed

Directions:

1. Organize the asparagus n a lined baking sheet, include the pesto and the other components, toss, bake at 400 degrees F within twenty mins.
2. Serve as a side dish.

Per serving: Calories: 114kcal; Protein: 2.6g; Carbs: 4.5g; Fat: 10.7g

111. Mascarpone Couscous

Preparation time: fifteen mins
Cooking time: seven and half hrs
Servings: four
Ingredients:

- one teacup couscous
- three and half teacups chicken stock
- half teacup mascarpone
- one tsp salt
- one tsp ground paprika

Directions:

1. Inside a saucepan, combine the chicken stock and the mascarpone, and then raise the mixture to a boil.
2. Include salt and ground paprika. Cook for one min while giving the mixture a gentle stir.
3. Take out the broth from the temp. and stir in the couscous prior to serving. After a thorough mixing, replace the cover.
4. Let the couscous sit undisturbed for ten mins.
5. Prior to serving, give the finished side dish a thorough stir.

Per serving: Calories: 227kcal; Protein: 9.7g; Carbs: 35.4g; Fat: 4.9g

112. Balsamic Cabbage

Preparation time: ten mins
Cooking time: twenty mins
Servings: four
Ingredients:

- one lb. green cabbage, roughly shredded
- two tbsps olive oil
- A tweak of black pepper
- one shallot, severed
- two garlic pieces, crushed
- two tbsps balsamic vinegar
- two tsps hot paprika
- one tsp sesame seeds

Directions:

1. Warm up a pot with the oil in a middling temp., include the shallot and the garlic, and sauté for five mins.
2. Include the cabbage and the other components, toss, cook at middling temp. for fifteen mins, split among plates and serve.

Per serving: Calories: 100kcal; Protein: 1.8g; Carbs: 8.2g; Fat: 7.5g

113. Spiced Nuts

Preparation time: ten mins
Cooking time: ten-fifteen mins
Servings: two
Ingredients:

- half teacup walnuts
- one teacup almonds
- one tsp ground turmeric
- quarter teacup sunflower seeds
- quarter teacup pumpkin puree
- quarter tsp garlic powder
- half tsp ground cumin
- quarter tsp red pepper flakes

Directions:

1. Put the oven on to preheat at 350 degrees Fahrenheit.
2. Blend the entire components in a mixing container, and then take out a baking sheet. Cook the nuts for ten-fifteen mins after spreading them out in a single layer on the baking pan.
3. Allow it to cool completely prior to putting it away.

Per serving: Calories: 180kcal; Protein: 3g; Carbs: 20g; Fat: 1g

114. Parmesan Endives

Preparation time: ten mins
Cooking time: twenty mins
Servings: four
Ingredients:

- four endives, shared lengthwise
- one tbsp lemon juice
- one tbsp lemon zest, grated
- two tbsps fat-free parmesan, grated
- two tbsps olive oil
- A tweak of black pepper

Directions:

1. In a baking dish, blend the endives with the lemon juice and the other components excluding the parmesan and toss.
2. Sprinkle the parmesan on top, bake the endives at 400 deg. F for twenty mins, and serve.

Per serving: Calories: 71kcal; Protein: 0.9g; Carbs: 2.2g; Fat: 7.1g

115. Fresh Strawberry Salsa

Preparation time: ten mins
Cooking time: zero mins
Servings: six-eight
Ingredients:

- half tsp lime zest, grated
- two tsps pure raw honey
- two kiwi fruit, skinned, severed
- half teacup fresh cilantro
- quarter teacup fresh lime juice
- two lbs. fresh ripe strawberries, hulled, severed
- half teacup red onion, finely severed
- one-two jalapeños, desowed, finely severed

Directions:

1. Include lime juice, lime zest and honey into a big container and whisk thoroughly.
2. Include remaining components then mix thoroughly. Cover and put away for a while for the flavors to set in. Serve.

Per serving: Calories: 119kcal; Protein: 9.2g; Carbs: 11.7g; Fat: 4.3g

116. Roasted Carrots

Preparation time: ten mins
Cooking time: forty mins
Servings: four
Ingredients:

- one onion, skinned & cut
- eight carrots, skinned & cut
- one tsp thyme, severed
- two tbsps of extra-virgin olive oil
- half tsp rosemary, severed
- quarter tsp ground pepper
- half tsp salt

Directions:

1. Set your oven to a temp. of 425° Fahrenheit.
2. Combine the carrots and onions by throwing them in a container with the thyme, rosemary, black pepper, and salt. Distribute out on the baking tray you have.
3. Roast for forty mins. Onions and carrots ought to be browned and cooked through at this point.

Per serving: Calories: 126kcal; Protein: 2g; Carbs: 16g; Fat: 6g

117. Beet Hummus

Preparation time: five mins
Cooking time: zero mins
Servings: two
Ingredients:

- one piece of garlic
- one skinless roasted beet
- one and three-quarter teacups of chickpeas
- half teacup of olive oil
- two tbsps of sunflower seeds
- Juice of one lemon
- quarter tsp of chili flakes
- one and half tsps of cumin
- one tsp of curry
- one tsp of maple syrup
- half tsp of oregano
- half tsp of salt
- one nub of fresh ginger

Directions:

1. Place every one of the ingredients in a blender and process until the mixture is completely smooth. Sprinkle with sunflower seeds prior to serving.
2. Relish!

Per serving: Calories: 423kcal; Protein: 13.9g; Carbs: 40.1g; Fat: 24.2g

118. Celery and Fennel Salad with Cranberries

Preparation time: fifteen mins
Cooking time: zero mins
Servings: six
Ingredients:

- quarter teacup extra-virgin olive oil
- two tbsps freshly squeezed lemon juice
- one tbsp Dijon mustard
- two teacups sliced celery
- half teacup severed fennel
- half teacup dried cranberries
- one tbsp crushed celery leaves

Directions:

1. In a serving container, pincludele the olive oil, lemon juice, and mustard.
2. Include the celery, fennel, and cranberries to the dressing and toss to coat. Sprinkle with the celery leaves and serve.

Per serving: Calories: 130kcal; Protein: 1g; Carbs: 13g; Fat: 9g

119. Roasted Garlic Chickpeas

Preparation time: five mins
Cooking time: twenty mins
Servings: two
Ingredients:

- four teacups cooked chickpeas, washed, drained & dried
- one tsp garlic powder
- one tsp sea salt
- Black pepper as required
- two tbsps olive oil

Directions:

1. Warm up your oven to 400°F before proceeding.
2. Pour the olive oil over the chickpeas and lay them out in a single layer on a baking tray.
3. Place in oven for twenty mins, mixing once at the ten-minute mark, and bake until golden brown.
4. Transfer the hot chickpeas to a container, then season them prior to placing them in a container with a tight-fitting lid. They can be stored at room temp. for a maximum of two days without losing their freshness.

Per serving: Calories: 150kcal; Protein: 4g; Carbs: 2g; Fat: 2g

120. Roasted Parsnips

Preparation time: five mins
Cooking time: thirty mins
Servings: four
Ingredients:

- one tbsp of extra-virgin olive oil
- two lbs. parsnips
- one tsp of kosher salt
- one-half tsp of Italian flavouring
- Severed parsley for garnishing

Directions:

1. Set your oven to a temp. of 400° Fahrenheit.
2. Take out the peel from the parsnips. Cube them into pieces that are one inch in size.
3. Next, add the seasoning, salt, and oil to a container, and whisk to combine.
4. Distribute this mixture across your baking tray. It ought to be done in a single layer.
5. Roast for a total of half an hour. Each ten mins, give it a stir.
6. Place on a plate and set aside. Dress the dish with chopped parsley.

Per serving: Calories: 124kcal; Protein: 2g; Carbs: 20g; Fat: 4g

121. Crispy Corn

Preparation time: eight mins
Cooking time: five mins
Servings: three
Ingredients:

- one teacup corn kernels
- one tbsp coconut flour
- half tsp salt
- three tbsps canola oil
- half tsp ground paprika
- three-quarter tsp chili pepper
- one tbsp water

Directions:

1. Place corn kernels, salt, and coconut flour in the mixing basin and stir to incorporate.
2. After the water has been added, thoroughly combine the corn with the spoon.
3. Include the canola oil to the pan and set it over medium temp.
4. After adding the corn kernel mixture, roast the mixture for four mins. Make sure to give it a stir every so often.
5. Once the corn kernels have reached the desired level of crunchiness, transfer them to a plate and help them dry using paper towels.
6. Include chile pepper and ground paprika. Toss everything together thoroughly.

Per serving: Calories: 179kcal; Protein: 2.1g; Carbs: 11.3g; Fat: 15g

122. Easy Guacamole

Preparation time: ten mins
Cooking time: zero mins
Servings: three
Ingredients:

- four avocados, shared & pitted
- one tsp garlic powder
- half tsp sea salt

Directions:

1. Using a spoon, remove the flesh from the avocado and place it within a container.
2. While continuing to mash, include your salt and garlic powder and continue to do so till the mixture is smooth. It will stay edible for up to two days if stored in the refrigerator.

Per serving: Calories: 358kcal; Protein: 7.2g; Carbs: 13.3g; Fat: 32.3g

123. Lima Beans Dish

Preparation time: ten mins
Cooking time: five hrs
Servings: ten
Ingredients:

- one green bell pepper, severed
- one sweet red pepper, severed
- one and half teacups tomato sauce, salt-free
- one yellow onion, severed
- half teacup of water
- sixteen oz. canned kidney beans, no-salt-included, drained and washed
- sixteen oz. canned black-eyed peas, no-salt-included, drained and washed
- fifteen oz. corn
- fifteen oz. canned lima beans, no-salt-included, drained and washed
- fifteen oz canned black beans, no-salt-included, drained
- two celery ribs, severed
- two bay leaves
- one tsp ground mustard
- one tbsp cider vinegar

Directions:

1. Combine the tomato sauce, celery, onion, green bell pepper, water, dried bay leaves, red pepper, vinegar, mustard, kidney beans, corn, black-eyed peas, and lima beans in your slow cooker. Cook on Low for about five hrs.
2. Throw away the bay leaves, then split the remaining mixture amongst four dishes and serve.

Per serving: Calories: 602kcal; Protein: 33g; Carbs: 117.7g; Fat: 4.8g

124. Cashew "Humus"

Preparation time: ten mins
Cooking time: zero mins
Servings: one
Ingredients:

- one teacup cashews, raw & soaked in water for fifteen mins & drained
- two pieces garlic
- quarter teacup water
- one tbsp olive oil
- one tsp lemon juice, fresh
- two tsps coconut aminos
- half tsp ground ginger
- Tweak of cayenne pepper
- quarter tsp sea salt, fine

Directions:

1. Combine every one of the components inside a blender, ensuring to scrape down the sides as needed. Keep blending it till it reaches a smooth consistency, and afterwards chill it in the refrigerator prior to serving.

Per serving: Calories: 112kcal; Protein: 2.1g; Carbs: 5.4g; Fat: 8.6g

125. Apple Crisp

Preparation time: fifteen mins
Cooking time: twenty-five mins
Servings: six-eight
Ingredients:
Topping:

- one and half teacups old-fashioned rolled oats
- two-third teacup shredded, unsweetened coconut
- one tsp salt
- half teacup stevia
- one-third teacup almond meal
- quarter tsp ground nutmeg
- two tsps ground cinnamon
- one teacup nuts, coarsely severed
- three tbsps dissolved coconut oil.

Apple filling:

- ten tart apples
- half teacup stevia
- two tbsps fresh-squeezed lemon juice
- one tbsp ground cinnamon
- quarter teacup arrowroot flour
- quarter tsp salt
- three tbsps dissolved coconut oil
- one tsp vanilla
- The zest of one orange

Directions:

1. Warm up the oven to 350 degrees Fahrenheit and then oil a baking pot that is nine inches by thirteen inches with coconut oil.
2. Inside a container, combine all of the topping components, then give it a good stir and put it away.
3. Inside a 2nd big basin, mix together all of the components for the filling, excluding the apples.
4. If you choose, you can keep the apple skins on the apples. Take out the core, then slice them extremely thinly (about one-eighth of an inch dense).
5. To get a uniform coating, whisk the apples in the components for the fillings. Put the apple combination in a baking dish, then distribute the topping over it and squash it down tightly. Bake the crisp until the topping is golden brown.
6. Put the dish in the oven and make sure there is a pot below it to catch any drippings.
7. Place the dish in the oven and bake for twenty-five mins, or till the topping is golden brown and the liquids are boiling. Apples ought to have a yielding texture.
8. Allow to mildly cool on a stand prior to serving.

Per serving: Calories: 446kcal; Protein: 6.1g; Carbs: 57.4g; Fat: 27.3g

Chapter 6. Snacks, Appetizers, Desserts, and Sweet Treats Recipes

126. Strawberry Granita 90
127. Fragrant Honey Panna Cotta 90
128. Honey Stewed Apples 91
129. Smashed Peas with Dill and Mint 91
130. Mango Mug Cake 91
131. Greek Yogurt with Berries, Nuts and Honey 91
132. Chocolate Cups 92
133. Cinnamon Turmeric Golden Milk 92
134. Cherry Vanilla Ice Cream 93
135. Ruby Pears Delight 93
136. Garlicky Dill Cucumber and Yogurt Dip 93
137. Fresh Blackberry Granita with Lemon Syrup 94
138. Chickpea Paste with Onion 94
139. Chickpea and Garlic Hummus 94
140. Skewers of Tofu and Zucchini 94
141. Pear and Cinnamon Pudding 95
142. Healthy Trail Mix 95
143. Sweet Potato Muffins 96
144. Coconut Rice with Blueberries 96
145. Stone Fruit Cobbler 97
146. Whole meal Rice Pudding with Plums 97
147. Sorbet with Honey and Goji Berries 98
148. Peanut Butter Toast with Vegetables 98
149. Citrus Spinach 98
150. Coconut Vanilla Tart 99

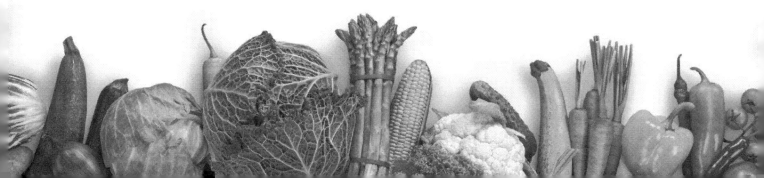

126. Strawberry Granita

Preparation time: two hrs
Cooking time: zero mins
Servings: four-six
Ingredients:

- one teacup water
- half teacup raw cane sugar
- half teacup lime juice
- 1 lb. strawberries, stems removed

Directions:

1. Fill a container with ice water. Mix the one teacup sugar and water inside a saucepot, dissolve the sugar with low heat.
2. Take out the syrup from the heat, put the pan in the ice-water bath, stir chill rapidly, then refrigerate the syrup 3 hours.
3. Reserve four to six strawberries for garnish. Organize the remaining strawberries inside a mixer. Blend 'til smooth, strain through a fine-mesh sieve into a container to remove the seeds.
4. Include the lime juice and half teacup of the simple syrup to the strawberry juice. Stir and taste.
5. Pour the strawberry solution into a thirteen-by-nine-by-two-in metal baking pot. Freeze about twenty-five mins.
6. Using a fork, stir the icy portions into the middle of the pan. Continue this process of mixing the icy edges into center every twenty-five mins about 1½ hours. Cover and freeze about 1 day.
7. Scrape the granita into containers, garnish with the reserved berries.
8. Enjoy.

Per serving: Calories: 44kcal; Protein: 0.6g; Carbs: 11.6g; Fat: 0.2g

127. Fragrant Honey Panna Cotta

Preparation time: ten mins
Cooking time: five mins
Servings: 6
Ingredients:

- two and half teacups canned unsweetened coconut milk
- two tsps gelatin
- quarter teacup honey
- one vanilla bean, split and seeds scraped
- Kosher salt

Blackberry-Lime Sauce

- two teacups blackberries
- one tsp raw cane sugar
- Zest of ½ lime, grated, plus two tsps lime juice

Directions:

1. Organize half teacup of coconut milk in a container. Sprinkle the gelatin over the top, sit for almost two mins.
2. Organize the remaining two teacups coconut milk, bean and its seeds, honey, and a tweak of salt in your saucepan. Warm at low temp., whisk till bubbles form take out from the temp. then let the solution steep for five mins.
3. Pour milk solution through a fine-mesh strainer into a container, discard the vanilla bean.
4. Whisk well the gelatin solution into the warm coconut solution. Split six ½-cup ramekins. Cover and refrigerate about four hrs.
5. To make the blackberry-lime sauce: Place the remaining components inside a moderate container. Using a fork gently mash the berries, leaving some large pieces of berry. Set aside for at least ten mins.

Per serving: Calories: 357kcal; Protein: 3.5g; Carbs: 37.8g; Fat: 24g

128. Honey Stewed Apples

Preparation time: five mins
Cooking time: five mins
Servings: four
Ingredients:

- two tbsps honey
- one tsp cinnamon, ground
- half tsp cloves, ground
- 4 apples

Directions:

1. Include the entire components to the inner pot. Now, pour in ⅓ C. of water.
2. Make sure the cover is tight. To cook at high pressure for two mins, select the "Manual" setting on your pressure cooker. When the cooking process is finished, perform a rapid pressure release, and then gently take off the cover.
3. Serve in individual containers. Bon appétit!

Per serving: Calories: 128kcal; Protein: 0g; Carbs: 34g; Fat: 0g

129. Smashed Peas with Dill and Mint

Preparation time: ten mins
Cooking time: eight-ten mins
Servings: four
Ingredients:

- four teacups frozen peas, thawed
- quarter teacup extra-virgin olive oil
- quarter teacup fresh dill, severed
- quarter teacup fresh mint, severed
- one tsp salt, plus includeitional as needed

Directions:

1. Place 2 inches of water in a pot, insert a steamer basket. Raise to a boil at high temp.
2. Place the peas in the basket. Cover then cook for eight-ten mins, or 'til the peas are bright green and soft. Drain and transfer to a blending container.
3. Mix in the olive oil, dill, mint, and salt to the blending container. Process till completely smooth, or pulse a few times and leave some texture.
4. Taste the solution then adjust the flavouring if needed.

Per serving: Calories: 243kcal; Protein: 9g; Carbs: 25g; Fat: 13g

130. Mango Mug Cake

Preparation time: five mins
Cooking time: ten mins
Servings: two
Ingredients:

- one medium-sized mango, skinned and cubed
- 2 eggs
- one tsp vanilla
- quarter tsp nutmeg, grated
- one tbsp cocoa powder
- two tbsps honey
- half teacup coconut flour

Directions:

1. Blend the coconut flour, eggs, honey, vanilla, nutmeg, and cocoa powder in 2 lightly greased mugs.
2. Then, include one teacup of water and a metal trivet to the Instant Pot. Lower the uncovered mugs onto the trivet.
3. Put the cover on tight. Select the "Manual" option, then set the pressure to high, and cook for ten mins. When the cooking process is finished, perform a rapid pressure release, and then gently take off the cover.
4. Top with cubed mango and serve chilled. Enjoy!

Per serving: Calories: 268kcal; Protein: 10g; Carbs: 34g; Fat: 10g

131. Greek Yogurt with Berries, Nuts and Honey

Preparation time: five mins

Cooking time: zero mins
Servings: four
Ingredients:

- one and half teacups blueberries
- three teacups unsweetened plain Greek yogurt
- half teacup honey
- three-quarter teacup severed mixed nuts

Directions:
1. Spoon the yogurt into four containers.
2. Sprinkle the nuts and blueberries over the yogurt, then drizzle with the honey.
3. Serve immediately.

Per serving: Calories: 457kcal; Protein: 15g; Carbs: 62g; Fat: 18g

132. Chocolate Cups

Preparation time: two hrs
Cooking time: zero mins
Servings: six
Ingredients:

- half teacup avocado oil
- one teacup chocolate, dissolved
- one tsp matcha powder
- three tbsps stevia

Directions:
1. Inside a dish, combine the chocolate, oil, and the remaining components. Using a whisk, thoroughly combine the mixture. Next, split the mixture into teacups and place in the freezer for two hrs prior to serving.

Per serving: Calories: 174kcal; Protein: 2g; Carbs: 3g; Fat: 9g

133. Cinnamon Turmeric Golden Milk

Preparation time: fifteen mins or fewer
Cooking time: three-four hrs on low
Servings: four to six
Ingredients:

- two tbsps coconut oil
- one (2-inch) piece fresh ginger, roughly severed
- four teacups unsweetened almond milk
- 4 cinnamon sticks
- 1 (4-inch) piece turmeric root, roughly severed
- one tsp raw honey, plus more as required

Directions:
1. Include the coconut oil, ginger, almond milk, cinnamon sticks and turmeric into the slow cooker, blend them together.
2. Cover the cooker then cook on low for three-four hrs.
3. Set a fine-mesh sieve over a clean container, pour in the contents of the cooker, discard the solids.
4. Include raw honey as required, start with one tsp.

Per serving: Calories: 133kcal; Protein: 1g; Carbs: 10g; Fat: 11g

134. Cherry Vanilla Ice Cream

Preparation time: ten mins
Cooking time: zero mins
Servings: four-six
Ingredients:

- one (ten oz.) package frozen no-included-sugar cherries
- three teacups unsweetened almond milk
- half tsp almond extract
- one tsp vanilla extract

Directions:

1. Include the cherries, almond milk, almond extract, and vanilla extract into your blender or blending container, blend 'til frequently homogenous; a few chunks of cherries are fine.
2. In a container with an airtight lid, pour the solution. Place into freezer and freeze thoroughly prior to serving.

Per serving: Calories: 82kcal; Protein: 1g; Carbs: 14gm; Fat: 2gm

135. Ruby Pears Delight

Preparation time: ten mins
Cooking time: ten mins
Servings: four
Ingredients:

- four pears
- 26 oz. grape juice
- 11 oz. currant jelly
- 4 garlic cloves
- Juice and zest of one lemon
- 4 peppercorns
- 2 rosemary springs
- ½ vanilla bean

Directions:

1. Pour the jelly and grape juice in your instant pot and mix with lemon zest and juice
2. In the mix, dip each pear and wrap them in a clean tin foil and place them orderly in the steamer basket of your instant pot
3. Blend peppercorns, rosemary, garlic cloves, and vanilla bean to the juice solution,
4. Seal the cover and cook at High for ten mins.
5. Release the pressure quickly, and carefully open the cover; bring out the pears, remove wrappers and arrange them on plates. Serve when cold with toppings of cooking juice.

Per serving: Calories: 145kcal; Protein: 1g; Carbs: 1g; Fat: 5g

136. Garlicky Dill Cucumber and Yogurt Dip

Preparation time: fifteen mins
Cooking time: one min
Servings: four
Ingredients:

- two tbsps extra-virgin olive oil
- one cucumber, skinned and shredded
- one teacup plain coconut yogurt
- one garlic piece, crushed
- one scallion, severed
- two tbsps severed fresh dill
- one tsp salt
- two tbsps freshly squeezed lemon juice

Directions:

1. In a fine-mesh strainer, include the shredded cucumber and drain it.
2. Include the yogurt, garlic, scallion, dill, salt, and lemon juice into a small container, stir them together.
3. Stir in the drained cucumber, then transfer them into a serving container.
4. Spray with the olive oil prior to serving.

Per serving: Calories: 104kcal; Protein: 1g; Carbs: 7g; Fat: 9g

137. Fresh Blackberry Granita with Lemon Syrup

Preparation time: ten mins plus four hrs to freeze
Cooking time: 0
Servings: four
Ingredients:

- half teacup raw honey
- one lb. fresh blackberries
- quarter teacup freshly squeezed lemon juice
- one tsp severed fresh thyme
- half teacup water

Directions:

1. Include the honey, blackberries, lemon juice, thyme and water into a blending container, process till puréed.
2. Set a fine-mesh sieve over an eight by eight inch metal baking dish, pour in the purée, discard the seeds. Transfer the baking dish into the freezer for two hrs. Take out the dish and stir the granita to break up any frozen sections, scraping along the sides. Place back to the freezer for 1 hour. Stir and scrape again. Place the solution back to the freezer till completely frozen, about four hrs total.
3. Cover the granita. When you serve, scrape off portions with a fork.

Per serving: Calories: 182kcal; Protein: 2g; Carbs: 46g; Fat: 1g

138. Chickpea Paste with Onion

Preparation time: fifteen mins, plus thirty mins to sit
Cooking time: 0
Servings: two teacups
Ingredients:

- one (15 oz.) can chickpeas, drained, washed
- quarter teacup extra-virgin olive oil
- quarter teacup fresh lemon juice
- quarter teacup crushed onion
- half tsp ground cumin
- one garlic piece, crushed
- one tsp sea salt
- quarter tsp red pepper flakes

Directions:

1. Inside a container, mash the chickpeas with a potato masher till mostly broken up.
2. Blend the olive oil, lemon juice, cumin, onion, garlic, salt and red pepper flakes, continue mash till a slightly chunky paste form.
3. Set aside about thirty mins at room temp. for the flavors to develop.
4. Enjoy.

Per serving: Calories: 110kcal; Protein: 3g; Carbs: 10g; Fat: 8g

139. Chickpea and Garlic Hummus

Preparation time: five mins
Cooking time: zero mins
Servings: 6
Ingredients:

- three garlic pieces, crushed
- two tbsps extra-virgin olive oil
- two tbsps tahini
- one (fourteen oz.) can chickpeas, drained
- Juice of one lemon
- half tsp sea salt
- Paprika, for garnish

Directions:

1. Inside a suitable mixer, blend the garlic, olive oil, tahini, chickpeas, lemon juice, and salt.
2. Blend till smooth.
3. Garnish as desired.

Per serving: Calories: 134kcal; Protein: 3.6g; Carbs: 8.6g; Fat: 10.8g

140. Skewers of Tofu and Zucchini

Preparation time: five mins
Cooking time: five mins
Servings: 6
Ingredients:

- 7 ounces grams of smoked tofu
- two courgettes
- two tbsps of olive oil
- one tweak of salt
- one tweak of red pepper

Directions:
1. Cut the tofu into cubes and brown it for five mins in a non-stick pan with a tablespoon of oil.
2. Cut the courgettes into slices, and with the help of a kitchen brush, grease them with the oil previously mixed with the salt and chili pepper.
3. Grill the courgettes without letting them burn.
4. Place a cube of tofu alternating with a slice of courgette on a skewer toothpick, repeat.
5. Continue till all components are consumed.

Per serving: Calories: 127kcal; Protein: 8g; Carbs: 4g; Fat: 9g

141. Pear and Cinnamon Pudding

Preparation time: ten mins
Cooking time: zero mins
Servings: two
Ingredients:

- 2 pears
- three-quarter teacup of low-fat cottage cheese
- one organic lemon
- one tbsp of maple syrup
- one tbsp of ground cinnamon
- one tbsp of severed hazelnuts

Directions:
1. Peel the pears and dice them, squeeze the lemon juice and put it in a container with the pears.
2. Include the syrup and mix thoroughly. Split the solution into two glasses and cover with the cottage cheese. Decorate with severed hazelnuts.

Per serving: Calories: 115kcal; Protein: 1g; Carbs: 31g; Fat: 0g

142. Healthy Trail Mix

Preparation time: five mins
Cooking time: zero mins
Servings: 12 to 14
Ingredients:

- one teacup sunflower seeds
- one teacup pumpkin seeds
- one teacup dried cranberries
- one teacup raisins
- one teacup large coconut flakes
- half teacup cacao nibs (optional)

Directions:
1. Include the sunflower seeds, pumpkin seeds, cranberries, raisins, coconut, and cacao nibs (if using) to a big container, stir them together.
2. Place the solution into large jars, store covered in a cool, dry place. Or portion into small containers for a quick grab-and-go option.

Per serving: Calories: 183kcal; Protein: 5g; Carbs: 19g; Fat: 11g

143. Sweet Potato Muffins

Preparation time: fifteen mins
Cooking time: twenty to twenty-five mins
Servings: twelve
Ingredients:

- one teacup sweet potato, cooked & pureed
- one and half teacups rolled oats
- one tsp baking powder
- half tsp baking soda
- one-third teacup coconut sugar
- one teacup almond milk
- quarter teacup almond butter
- one egg
- two tbsps olive oil
- one tsp ground cinnamon
- one tsp vanilla extract, pure
- quarter tsp sea salt

Directions:

1. Warm up your oven to 375 degrees Fahrenheit before proceeding.
2. Prepare your muffin tray by placing paper liners in it, and have a blending container ready.
3. Pulse your oats till it produces a course flour. It should first be placed in a small container after which it should be put aside.
4. Inside a blender, combine the entire of your components, with the exception of the oat flour, and mix till homogeneous.
5. While the machine is running, gradually put in your oat flour and pulse it till it is completely blended.
6. Divide the batter among the prepared cupcake tins, and bake for twenty to twenty-five mins. Prior to serving, you should wait a minimum of five mins for them to cool off.

Per serving: Calories: 143kcal; Protein: 6g; Carbs: 1g; Fat: 3g

144. Coconut Rice with Blueberries

Preparation time: ten mins
Cooking time: thirty mins
Servings: four
Ingredients:

- one teacup brown basmati rice
- 2 dates, pitted and severed
- one teacup coconut milk
- one tsp sea salt
- one teacup water
- quarter teacup toasted slivered almonds
- half teacup shaved coconut
- one teacup fresh blueberries

Directions:

1. Blend the basmati rice, dates, coconut milk, salt, and water in a saucepan. Stir to mix thoroughly. Raise to a boil.
2. Decrease its temp. to low, then simmer for thirty mins or till the rice is soft.
3. Split them into four containers and serve with almonds, coconut, and blueberries on top.

Per serving: Calories: 397kcal; Protein: 6.6g; Carbs: 50.8g; Fat: 20g

145. Stone Fruit Cobbler

Preparation time: ten mins
Cooking time: twenty mins
Servings: eight
Ingredients:

- one tsp coconut oil plus quarter teacup dissolved
- two teacups sliced fresh peaches
- two teacups sliced fresh nectarines
- two tbsps lemon juice
- three-quarter teacup almond flour
- three-quarter teacup rolled oats
- quarter teacup coconut sugar
- one tsp ground cinnamon
- half tsp vanilla extract
- Dash salt
- Filtered water for mixing

Directions:

1. At 425 degrees F, preheat your oven.
2. Coat the bottom of a suitable cast-iron griddle with one tsp of coconut oil.
3. In the griddle, mix the peaches, nectarines, and lemon juice.
4. In a suitable blending container or mixer, include the almond flour, oats, coconut sugar, quarter teacup of dissolved coconut oil, cinnamon, vanilla, and salt. Pulse till the oats are broken up, and the solution resembles a dry dough.
5. Pour the dough into a suitable container. With your fingers, break the dough into large chunks and spray across the top of the fruit.
6. Bake the food for twenty mins. Serve warm.

Per serving: Calories: 110kcal; Protein: 3.1g; Carbs: 17.8g; Fat: 3.4g

146. Whole meal Rice Pudding with Plums

Preparation time: ten mins
Cooking time: twenty-five mins
Servings: three
Ingredients:

- one teacup of brown rice
- four teacups of oat milk
- one tbsp of maple syrup
- one tweak of salt
- one tsp of vanilla extract
- 2 organic eggs
- 5 dried and pitted plums

Directions:

1. Put the rice in the oat milk with the vanilla, salt, syrup inside a saucepot and cook at low temp.
2. Stir often. Cook till the milk is completely immersed and the rice is soft. Take out from fire.
3. Beat eggs. Coarsely chop the plums.
4. Incorporate the eggs into the rice, include the prunes and return to the heat at low temp. for one min.

Per serving: Calories: 337kcal; Protein: 10g; Carbs: 6g; Fat: 14g

147. Sorbet with Honey and Goji Berries

Preparation time: fifteen mins + 1sixty mins waiting time
Cooking time: zero mins
Servings: two
Ingredients:

- five tablespoons of raw honey
- three tbsps of goji berries
- one teacup of water

Directions:

1. Soak the goji berries for almost thirty mins, drain well. Bring the cup of water to a boil and dissolve the honey.
2. Allow to cool and include the goji berries.
3. Place in a container and place in the freezer for almost thirty mins.
4. Take out from the freezer, mix thoroughly and put it back in the freezer for thirty mins.
5. Repeat 5 times.

Per serving: Calories: 175kcal; Protein: 0g; Carbs: 47g; Fat: 0g

148. Peanut Butter Toast with Vegetables

Preparation time: ten mins
Cooking time: zero mins
Servings: two
Ingredients:

- four slices of whole meal toast bread
- one tbsp of peanut butter
- 1 cucumber
- one onion
- 1 tomato
- one tbsp of severed fresh basil

Directions:

1. Toast the toast slices without burning them, spread the peanut butter on two slices.
2. Skin the cucumber and cut it into slices, chop the onion, wash and slice the tomato.
3. Put the cucumber slices on top of the buttered bread slices, include the tomato slices, the severed onion and close the toast with the other slices of bread.

Per serving: Calories: 220kcal; Protein: 8g; Carbs: 35g; Fat: 5g

149. Citrus Spinach

Preparation time: ten mins
Cooking time: seven mins
Servings: four
Ingredients:

- two tbsps extra-virgin olive oil
- four teacups fresh baby spinach
- two garlic pieces, crushed
- Juice of ½ orange
- Zest of ½ orange
- half tsp sea salt
- one-eighth tsp black pepper

Directions:

1. In a suitable griddle at medium-high temp., heat the olive oil till it shimmers.
2. Toss in the spinach and cook for three mins, blending irregularly.
3. Include the garlic. Cook for thirty secs, blending regularly.
4. Include the orange juice, orange zest, salt, and pepper. Cook for almost two mins, constantly mixing, till the juice evaporates.

Per serving: Calories: 117kcal; Protein: 2g; Carbs: 12.8g; Fat: 7.1g

150. Coconut Vanilla Tart

Preparation time: ten mins
Cooking time: fifteen mins
Servings: 16
Ingredients:

- two tbsps coconut oil
- two tbsps granulated erythritol or another low-carb sweetener
- one tsp pure vanilla extract
- one (thirteen and half oz.) tin low-fat coconut milk
- Tweak of of fine Himalayan salt
- Grated zest of 1 lime or lemon, plus more for garnish
- one tbsp unflavored grass-fed beef gelatin
- 1 pie crust, baked in an 8-inch springform pan
- two tbsps unsweetened shredded coconut, for garnish

Directions:

1. Melt the coconut oil in your small saucepot at middling temp. Stir in the erythritol and simmer for ten mins, till it dissolves into a syrup, blending irregularly.
2. Meanwhile, include the vanilla extract, coconut milk, salt and citrus zest into a small container, whisk them together.
3. Stir the coconut milk solution into the syrup very quickly. Cook till the solution is steaming, almost at a simmer, about 5 to eight mins. As you whisk vigorously, spray in the gelatin. Stir till it's fully dissolved.
4. Pour the coconut milk solution into the prepared crust slowly. Put the tart on a plate or tray in case anything seeps from the springform pan. Place in the fridge to chill for four hrs, or till the center is completely set.
5. Garnish with more grated citrus zest and shredded coconut and serve. Use plastic wrap to wrap the leftovers and store in your fridge for almost three days.

Per serving: Calories: 142kcal; Protein: 2.4g; Carbs: 4.4g; Fat: 13.5g

Chapter 7. 30 - Days Meal Plan

Day	Breakfast	Lunch	Dinner	Dessert
1	Overnight Coconut Chia Oats	Chicken Lettuce Cups	Seared Garlicky Coconut Scallops	Fragrant Honey Panna Cotta
2	Mushroom and Bell Pepper Omelet	Fresh Spring Roll Wraps	Pork Kabobs with Bell Peppers	Greek Yogurt with Berries, Nuts and Honey
3	Spiced Morning Chia Pudding	Cabbage with Anchovies	Spiced Ground Beef	Stone Fruit Cobbler
4	Buckwheat Waffles	Kale Cod Secret	Garlic Cod Meal	Honey Stewed Apples
5	Plum, Pear and Berry-Baked Brown Rice	Chicken with Snow Peas and Brown Rice	Pork with Thyme Sweet Potatoes	Smashed Peas with Dill and Mint
6	Coconut Pancakes	Easy Slow Cooker Caramelized Onions	Roasted Seasoned Carrots	Chickpea Paste with Onion
7	Gingerbread Oatmeal	Spicy Wasabi Mayonnaise	Ginger Carrot and Pineapple Juice	Mango Mug Cake
8	Spinach Frittata	Coconut-Crusted Shrimp	Pork with Olives	Chocolate Cups
9	Chia Breakfast Pudding	Stir-Fried Squash	Salmon Broccoli Bowl	Cinnamon Turmeric Golden Milk
10	Oatmeal Pancakes	Broccoli with Garlic and Lemon	Spiced Morning Chia Pudding	Fresh Blackberry Granita with Lemon Syrup
11	Yogurt, Berry, And Walnut Parfait	Pesto Portobello Mushroom Burger	Beef with Carrot & Broccoli	Sorbet with Honey and Goji Berries
12	Spiced Popcorn	Mushroom Tacos	Pork with Chili Zucchinis and Tomatoes	Coconut Rice with Blueberries
13	Poached Eggs	Curried Okra	Oregano Pork	Honey Scallops
14	Buckwheat Crêpes with Berries	Turmeric Endives	Seared Syrupy Sage Pork Patties	Peanut Butter Toast with Vegetables
15	Spinach Fritters	Stir-Fried Almond and Spinach	Pork with Thyme and Sage Sausage	Ruby Pears Delight
16	Smoked Salmon Scrambled Eggs	Sweet Potato Puree	Cranberry Pork	Chickpea and Garlic Hummus
17	Overnight Muesli	Roasted Portobellos With Rosemary	Chicken with Coconut Milk	Cherry Vanilla Ice Cream
18	Gingerbread Oatmeal	Stir-Fried Squash	Pork Kabobs with Bell Peppers	Fragrant Honey Panna Cotta

19	Buckwheat Lemon Tabbouleh	Mushroom Tacos	Roasted Chicken	Greek Yogurt with Berries, Nuts and Honey
20	Seared Syrupy Sage Pork Patties	Coconut Chili Salmon	Mustard Pork Mix	Smashed Peas with Dill and Mint
21	Mushroom and Bell Pepper Omelet	Sweet Potato Puree	Salmon Broccoli Bowl	Mango Mug Cake
22	Spiced Morning Chia Pudding	Sauté Lentil Sloppy Joes	Ginger Carrot and Pineapple Juice	Stone Fruit Cobbler
23	Oatmeal Pancakes	Roasted Seasoned Carrots	Garlic Cod Meal	Chickpea Paste with Onion
24	Yogurt, Berry, And Walnut Parfait	Baked Sweet Potatoes with Tomatoes	Pork with Olives	Chocolate Cups
25	Buckwheat Waffles	Onion and Orange Healthy Salad	Beef with Carrot & Broccoli	Fresh Blackberry Granita with Lemon Syrup
26	Spiced Popcorn	Mushroom Tacos	Spiced Ground Beef	Coconut Rice with Blueberries
27	Poached Eggs	Cilantro and Avocado Platter	Pork with Thyme Sweet Potatoes	Cinnamon Turmeric Golden Milk
28	Buckwheat Crêpes with Berries	Stir-Fried Almond and Spinach	Chicken with Snow Peas and Brown Rice	Sorbet with Honey and Goji Berries
29	Spiced Morning Chia Pudding	Stir-Fried Squash	Oregano Pork	Honey Stewed Apples
30	Overnight Coconut Chia Oats	Curried Okra	Seared Garlicky Coconut Scallops	Ruby Pears Delight

Chapter 8. Frequently Asked Questions (FAQs)

Q: What foods should I include in an anti-inflammatory diet?

A: An anti-inflammatory diet should include plenty of fruits & vegetables, especially those rich in antioxidants and phytochemicals, such as berries, leafy greens, and cruciferous vegetables. It should also incorporate whole grains, lean proteins (such as fish, poultry, legumes), healthy fats (like olive oil, avocados, nuts, and seeds), and herbs and spices known for their anti-inflammatory properties, such as turmeric, ginger, and garlic.

Q: Are there any foods I should avoid in an anti-inflammatory diet?

A: Yes, there are foods that are generally recommended to be avoided or minimized in an anti-inflammatory diet. These include processed foods, sugary snacks and beverages, refined carbohydrates (like white bread & pasta), fried foods, red and processed meats, and foods high in trans fats and saturated fats. It's also advisable to limit alcohol consumption and avoid or reduce intake of foods that you may have a personal sensitivity or allergy to.

Q: Can an anti-inflammatory diet help with weight loss?

A: Yes, an anti-inflammatory diet can be beneficial for weight loss. By focusing on whole, nutrient-dense foods and avoiding processed and high-calorie foods, it can help reduce calorie intake while providing essential nutrients. Additionally, some anti-inflammatory foods can boost metabolism and promote fat burning in the body, contributing to weight loss.

Q: Can I have coffee or caffeine while following an anti-inflammatory diet?

A: Moderate consumption of coffee or caffeine is generally acceptable on an anti-inflammatory diet. In fact, coffee contains antioxidants that may have anti-inflammatory properties. However, excessive consumption or added sweeteners and creamers can contribute to inflammation. It's best to consume coffee in moderation and choose healthier options like black coffee or adding a small amount of unsweetened plant-based milk.

Q: How long does it take to see the effects of an anti-inflammatory diet?

A: The time it takes to see the effects of an anti-inflammatory diet can vary depending on individual factors such as current health status, dietary habits, and lifestyle. Some people may start experiencing positive changes, such as improved digestion and increased energy, within a few weeks of adopting an anti-inflammatory diet. However, significant changes in inflammation markers and long-term health benefits may take several months or more of consistent adherence to the diet.

Q: Can I still enjoy occasional treats or cheat meals while following an anti-inflammatory diet?

A: While the goal of an anti-inflammatory diet is to prioritize whole, nutrient-dense foods, occasional treats or cheat meals can be enjoyed in moderation. It's important to maintain a balanced approach and not feel overly restricted, as strict and unsustainable diets can be difficult to follow long-term. However, it's best to make healthier choices for treats whenever possible, such as opting for dark chocolate or homemade desserts made with natural sweeteners instead of processed sugary treats.

Q: How can I navigate social situations while following an anti-inflammatory diet?

A: Navigating social situations while following an anti-inflammatory diet can be challenging, but with some planning and communication, it's possible to maintain your dietary preferences. Here are a few tips:

- Inform the host or organizer about your dietary restrictions. Offer to bring a dish that aligns with your diet to ensure there will be an option you can enjoy.
- Look for dishes composed of fresh fruits, vegetables, lean proteins, and whole grains. Avoid processed foods and excessive added sugars.
- Opt for salads, grilled proteins, and vegetable-based dishes. Fill your plate with these options and enjoy them mindfully.
- If there are limited options, bring your own healthy snacks or small meals to avoid going hungry or compromising your diet.

Q: What are some strategies for maintaining an anti-inflammatory diet while eating out at restaurants?

A: Here are some strategies for sticking to an anti-inflammatory diet while eating out:

- Look up the restaurant's menu online before going. This allows you to identify dishes that align with your dietary preferences and avoid last-minute unhealthy choices.
- Opt for dishes that are grilled, baked, or steamed, as these cooking methods generally use less added fats and are healthier choices. Avoid fried or breaded options.
- Don't hesitate to ask your server for modifications to suit your dietary needs. Ask for dressings or sauces on the side, substitute ingredients, or request extra vegetables instead of starchy sides.
- Look for dishes that are rich in vegetables and include lean protein sources like grilled chicken, fish, or legumes. Fill your plate with these anti-inflammatory options.
- Restaurant portions are often larger than necessary. Consider sharing a dish with a friend or ask for a to-go box and save half of the meal for later.

Q: How can I maintain an anti-inflammatory diet while traveling?

A: Here are some tips for maintaining an anti-inflammatory diet while traveling:

- Bring along snacks like fresh fruits, nuts, seeds, or homemade granola bars. These can be convenient options when healthy choices are limited.
- Visit local grocery stores or markets to stock up on fresh produce, lean proteins, and healthy snacks. You can prepare simple meals in your accommodation using these ingredients.
- Choose whole foods like salads, grilled proteins, vegetables, and whole grains whenever possible. Avoid highly processed and fried foods, which can contribute to inflammation.
- Learn about the local cuisine and identify dishes that are likely to be more aligned with an anti-inflammatory diet. Look for traditional dishes that include fresh ingredients and healthy cooking methods.
- Drink plenty of water to stay hydrated, as travel can be dehydrating. Adequate hydration helps maintain overall health and supports your body's natural anti-inflammatory processes.

Anti-Inflammatory Cookbook

Q: Are there any potential risks or side effects of following an anti-inflammatory diet?

A: In general, an anti-inflammatory diet is considered safe and beneficial for most individuals. However, if you have any underlying health conditions or specific dietary restrictions, it's important to consult with a healthcare professional or a registered dietitian before making significant changes to your diet. Additionally, some people may experience initial detoxification symptoms, such as headaches or fatigue, when transitioning to a healthier eating pattern, but these usually resolve within a few days.

Index

Ahi Poke with Cucumber; 62
Apple Crisp; 88
Avocado Side Salad; 32
Baked Sweet Potatoes with Tomatoes; 74
Balsamic Cabbage; 83
Basil Olives Mix; 82
Beef & Vegetable Soup; 33
Beef with Carrot & Broccoli; 46
Beet Hummus; 84
Braised Kale; 70
Broccoli with Garlic and Lemon; 78
Brown Rice and Chicken Soup; 31
Buckwheat Crêpes with Berries; 20
Buckwheat Lemon Tabbouleh; 65
Buckwheat Waffles; 21
Cabbage With Anchovies; 58
Cashew "Humus"; 87
Cauliflower Hash Brown; 69
Cauliflower Mashed Potatoes; 73
Celery and Fennel Salad with Cranberries; 85
Cherry Vanilla Ice Cream; 93
Chia Breakfast Pudding; 27
Chicken Lettuce Cups; 50
Chicken Noodle Soup; 38
Chicken Squash Soup; 39
Chicken with Coconut Milk; 50
Chicken with Snow Peas and Brown Rice; 51
Chickpea and Garlic Hummus; 94
Chickpea Paste with Onion; 94
Chili Broccoli; 80
Chipotle Squash Soup; 37
Chocolate Cups; 92
Chopped Tuna Salad; 39
Cilantro And Avocado Platter; 77
Cinnamon Chicken Pesto Pasta; 53
Cinnamon Turmeric Golden Milk; 92
Citrus Spinach; 98
Coconut Cashew Soup with Butternut Squash; 33
Coconut Chili Salmon; 59
Coconut Pancakes; 28
Coconut Rice with Blueberries; 96
Coconut Vanilla Tart; 99
Coconut-Crusted Shrimp; 63
Couscous Salad; 41
Cranberry Pork; 46
Crispy Beef Carnitas; 47

Crispy Corn; 86
Cucumber Bites; 22
Curried Okra; 68
Easy Guacamole; 86
Easy Slow Cooker Caramelized Onions; 75
Easy Turkey Lettuce Wraps; 51
Fennel Pear Soup; 40
Fish Sticks with Avocado Dipping Sauce; 61
Fragrant Honey Panna Cotta; 90
Fresh Blackberry Granita with Lemon Syrup; 94
Fresh Mussels in Coconut Herb Broth; 58
Fresh Spring Roll Wraps; 67
Fresh Strawberry Salsa; 84
Garbanzo and Kidney Bean Salad; 32
Garlic Cod Meal; 57
Garlicky Dill Cucumber and Yogurt Dip; 93
Ginger Carrot and Pineapple Juice; 65
Gingerbread Oatmeal; 25
Golden Mushroom Soup; 30
Greek Yogurt with Berries, Nuts and Honey; 91
Green Beans; 81
Healthy Trail Mix; 95
Herbed Mussels Treat; 60
Honey Scallops; 56
Honey Stewed Apples; 91
Italian Wedding Soup; 34
Kale Cod Secret; 59
Lemon Asparagus; 82
Lentils And Turmeric Soup; 31
Lima Beans Dish; 87
Lime Carrots; 80
Lime Spinach and Chickpeas Salad; 30
Mango Mug Cake; 91
Mascarpone Couscous; 82
Mushroom and Bell Pepper Omelet; 26
Mushroom Tacos; 68
Mustard Pork Mix; 44
Nutty and Fruity Garden Salad; 40
Oatmeal Pancakes; 18
Onion and Orange Healthy Salad; 78
Orange Chicken Legs; 52
Orange Soup; 36
Oregano Pork; 48
Overnight Coconut Chia Oats; 18
Overnight Muesli; 25
Paprika Brussels Sprouts; 73

Anti-Inflammatory Cookbook

Parmesan Endives; 83
Peanut Butter Toast With Vegetables; 98
Pear And Cinnamon Pudding; 95
Persimmon Salad; 34
Pesto Portobello Mushroom Burger; 66
Plum, Pear and Berry-Baked Brown Rice; 24
Poached Eggs; 23
Pork Kabobs with Bell Peppers; 44
Pork with Chili Zucchinis and Tomatoes; 48
Pork with Olives; 43
Pork with Thyme Sweet Potatoes; 43
Recipe for Ruby Pears Delight; 93
Roasted Carrot Soup; 38
Roasted Carrots; 84
Roasted Chicken; 54
Roasted Garlic Chickpeas; 85
Roasted Parsnips; 85
Roasted Portobellos With Rosemary; 76
Roasted Seasoned Carrots; 70
Rosemary Chicken; 53
Salmon Broccoli Bowl; 60
Salt & Vinegar Kale Crisps; 80
Sauté Lemon-Caper Trout; 57
Sauté Lentil Sloppy Joes; 66
Seared Garlicky Coconut Scallops; 56
Seared Syrupy Sage Pork Patties; 19
Shoepeg Corn Salad; 41
Skewers Of Tofu And Zucchini; 94
Smashed Peas with Dill and Mint; 91

Smoked Salmon Scrambled Eggs; 21
Sorbet With Honey And Goji Berries; 98
Soup Of Oysters And Mushrooms; 62
Southwestern Bean-And-Pepper Salad; 37
Spiced Ground Beef; 45
Spiced Morning Chia Pudding; 24
Spiced Nuts; 83
Spiced Popcorn; 23
Spicy Pumpkin Soup; 35
Spicy Wasabi Mayonnaise; 76
Spinach Frittata; 19
Spinach Fritters; 26
Stir-Fried Almond And Spinach; 76
Stir-Fried Squash; 67
Stone Fruit Cobbler; 97
Strawberry Granita; 90
Stuffed Pepper Soup; 35
Sweet Potato Muffins; 96
Sweet Potato Puree; 71
Tomato Bulgur; 81
Turkey Sausages; 52
Turkey with Thyme and Sage Sausage; 20
Turmeric Endives; 69
Vegetable Potpie; 77
Warm Chia-Berry Non-dairy Yogurt; 27
Wheatberry Salad; 36
Wholemeal Rice Pudding With Plums; 97
Yogurt, Berry, and Walnut Parfait; 22
Zucchini Arugula and Olive Salad; 75

Conversion Table

Volume Equivalents (Liquid)

US Standard	US Standard (ounces)	Metric (approximate)
two tbsps	1 fl. oz.	30 milliliter
quarter teacup	2 fl. oz.	60 milliliter
half teacup	4 fl. oz.	120 milliliter
one teacup	8 fl. oz.	240 milliliter
one and half teacups	12 fl. oz.	355 milliliter
two teacups or one pint	16 fl. oz.	475 milliliter
four teacups or one quart	32 fl. oz.	1 Liter
one gallon	128 fl. oz.	4 Liter

Volume Equivalents (Dry)

US Standard	Metric (approximate)
one-eighth tsp	0.5 milliliter
quarter tsp	1 milliliter
half tsp	2 milliliter
three-quarter tsp	4 milliliter
one tsp	5 milliliter
one tbsp	15 milliliter
quarter teacup	59 milliliter
one-third teacup	79 milliliter
half teacup	118 milliliter
two-third teacup	156 milliliter
three-quarter teacup	177 milliliter
one teacup	235 milliliter
two teacups or one pint	475 milliliter
three teacups	700 milliliter
four teacups or one quart	1 Liter

Oven Temperatures

Fahrenheit (F)	Celsius (C) (approximate)
250 deg.F	120 deg.C
300 deg.F	150 deg.C
325 deg.F	165 deg.C
350 deg.F	180 deg.C

375 deg.F	190 deg.C
400 deg.F	200 deg.C
425 deg.F	220 deg.C
450 deg.F	230 deg.C

Weight Equivalents

US Standard	Metric (approximate)
one tbsp	15 gm
half oz.	15 gm
one oz.	30 gm
two oz.	60 gm
four oz.	115 gm
eight oz.	225 gm
twelve oz.	340 gm
sixteen oz. or one lb.	455 gm

Conclusion

Inflammation is the body's natural response to infection, illness, and injury. It involves the production of white blood cells, immune system cells, and cytokines that help fight infections. Acute inflammation is characterized by redness, discomfort, heat, and swelling, while chronic inflammation may occur without noticeable symptoms. Chronic inflammation can be triggered or aggravated by factors such as obesity and stress. Blood markers like C-reactive protein, homocysteine, TNF alpha, and IL-6 can indicate inflammation.

For example, when you cut your finger, it becomes red and swollen due to inflammation. Knee injuries can also lead to swollen and inflamed knees. While some inflammation is beneficial for the healing process, excessive inflammation can contribute to various diseases. Chronic inflammation has been linked to conditions like cancer, heart disease, Alzheimer's disease, and depression.

Certain daily habits can trigger inflammation, especially if repeated over time. Consuming excessive amounts of sugar and high-fructose corn syrup is particularly harmful. Insulin resistance, which can result from these dietary factors, is associated with health issues like diabetes and obesity. Refined carbohydrate diets, including white bread, have been associated with inflammation, insulin resistance, and obesity. Trans fats found in processed and packaged foods can damage the endothelial cells lining the arteries. Many processed foods also contain vegetable oils, and imbalances in omega-6 and omega-3 fatty acids have been linked to increased inflammation.

In addition to diet, excessive alcohol consumption and high intake of processed meat can induce inflammation in the body. Sedentary behavior is another significant non-dietary risk factor for inflammation.

To reduce inflammation, it is recommended to consume fewer inflammatory foods and increase the intake of anti-inflammatory substances. Choosing whole, nutrient-dense foods that are high in antioxidants is preferable to processed foods. By following recipes that prioritize these principles, you can work towards achieving your health goals.

Made in the USA
Columbia, SC
25 September 2023